28 DAYS
TO READING
WITHOUT GLASSES

D0963915

28 DAYS
TO READING
WITHOUT GLASSES
A Natural Method for Improving Your Vision

LISETTE SCHOLL

Illustrations by Sarah C. Newberry

A CITADEL PRESS BOOK
Published by Carol Publishing Group

To Jim
who sees what's deep inside

A Citadel Press Book
Published by Carol Publishing Group
Citadel Press is a registered trademark of Carol Communications, Inc.

Editorial, sales and distribution, rights and permissions inquiries should be
addressed to Carol Publishing Group, 120 Enterprise Avenue, Secaucus, N.J.
07094.

In Canada: Canadian Manda Group, One Atlantic Avenue, Suite 105, Toronto,
Ontario, M6K 3E7

Carol Publishing Group books may be purchased in bulk at special discounts for
sales promotion, fund-raising, or educational purposes. Special editions can be
created to specifications. For details, contact Special Sales Department, Carol
Publishing Group, 120 Enterprise Avenue, Secaucus, N.J. 07094.

Manufactured in the United States of America
10 9 8 7 6 5 4 3 2 1

Library of Congress Cataloging-in-Publication Data

Scholl, Lisette.
    28 days to reading without glasses : a natural method for
improving your vision / Lisette Scholl.
        p.   cm.
    ISBN 0–8065–2059–0 (pbk.)
        1. Presbyopia—Alternative treatment.   2. Visual training.
3. Behavioral optometry.   4. Bates method of orthoptics.   I. Title.
RE938.5.S36   1998
617.7'55—dc21   98–24464
                                                                   CIP

CONTENTS

Acknowledgments   vii

Preface   ix

Introduction   3

Part One: The Program   15

Part Two: Future Vision   247

The Peace Pilgrim's Symptoms of Inner Peace   254

Recommended Reading   256

ACKNOWLEDGMENTS

Without the generous help of friends and loved ones this project would have been a long-delayed and formidable task.

A very special thanks goes to Wolfgang Gillessen, my colleague, longtime friend, and "angel." It was his initial encouragement and help that made this book a reality.

Finding the time and space for the writing was sometimes challenging. I am especially grateful for the Zurich hospitality (and moments of inspiration) of Drs. Tobias Kohler and Thomas Cotar. Here at home the patience and help of the Newberry family (Jim, Sarah, Grace, Joseph, Jacob, and Micah) often went beyond the call of duty.

Tish Cook, Kathy Johnston, and Brett Mitchell came through with invaluable moral support as well as practical hands on help.

Sarah Newberry created not only wonderful illustrations but was also a delightful work partner.

Above all, I thank my partner Jim Newberry. He gave me love, support, help, inspiration, insights, invaluable information, and kept me going with reenergizing bodywork sessions that are any writer's dream come true.

PREFACE

This book is for you if you:

- Have excellent near-point vision and want to keep it that way.
- Are developing "shortening of the arms"—you can't hold print far enough away to read it.
- Are one of nearly seventy-seven million people, mostly over forty, who suffer from presbyopia, an inability to focus sharply for near vision.
- Have noticed your ability to shift focus becoming sluggish, perhaps even a blurring at all distances.
- Use weak, moderate, or strong reading glasses, or even bifocals or trifocals.
- Have used these glasses for a short time or for many years.
- Have other visual conditions, such as myopia (nearsightedness), astigmatism, cataracts, glaucoma, or another condition.
- Experience eye strain, fatigue, or headaches when you read, or try to focus on that great vision nemesis—the computer screen.

Going through this program can bring any of the following changes in your vision:

- Complete freedom from reading glasses

- A need for glasses only under adverse conditions
- Visual skills that will get you through many adverse conditions and emergency situations
- A weaker prescription and greater independence from reading aids
- An improvement in any other visual condition
- A healthy, comfortable freedom from sunglasses, except when excessive glare makes them advisable
- Clearer night vision

I must warn you, however, that there are side effects to this program. As your vision improves, you may also experience:

- Less stress and more relaxation
- More energy
- Better health and fitness
- A more positive attitude and greater self-confidence
- Improved balance and hand-eye coordination
- Uncontrollable urges to laugh and have more fun in your life
- An inability to take things, including yourself, as seriously as before
- A new outlook on the whole concept of aging
- A slowing down and even reversal of your aging process

All this from a few eye exercises? Well, not exactly. This is a holistic program, because vision is a complex process influenced by our whole being. I've been helping people improve their eyesight for more than twenty years, and I've yet to work with anyone who has achieved significant and lasting improvement with eye exercises alone. Circulation, nutrition, physical activity, beliefs, attitudes, and other factors also play powerful roles in our visual perception. But don't despair, this isn't a monumental undertaking of life-altering proportions! It takes only some minor adjustments to your current lifestyle to have a major impact on your vision. This program is designed to take everything in small, gradual increments.

A few of you will make nearly instantaneous and dramatic leaps back into clarity, but most of us make these changes more gradually. This is especially true when it comes to aging eyes and visual skills. You'll be literally turning back the clock, and what took some time to degenerate usually takes some time to regenerate.

You may very well have been told that aging eyes can't be rejuvenated, but it's just not so. They have been traditionally regarded as isolated little machines that break down with time, but this is a misconception. Our eyes are just as responsive as the rest of our bodies to good care and exercise as a compensation for the toll of time.

Consider what would happen if you went to the doctor with stiffness, aches, and pains. Not too long ago you might have been given a cane and pain killers, but now you would more likely receive counseling on diet and exercise to improve your circulation and flexibility.

It's exactly the same situation with your eyesight. You can let it passively deteriorate and rely on increasingly strong crutches, or put it on a health and fitness program. We lay practitioners of vision improvement methods are not alone in this holistic approach. The ranks of highly trained "behavioral" optometrists are growing every day. You may want to enlist the aid of one. If you cannot find one, perhaps you'll play a part in bringing a traditional optometrist into the new way of looking at vision.

28 DAYS
TO READING
WITHOUT GLASSES

INTRODUCTION:
COMING BACK TO CLEAR

> We shall not cease from exploration
> And the end of all our exploring
> Will be to arrive where we started
> And know the place for the first time.
>
> T. S. Elliot

Have you talked to an eye doctor about the program you're about to embark on? If so, the odds are pretty overwhelming that it was scoffed at. Even if you're lucky enough to be going to one of the small (but growing!) number of behavioral optometrists practicing visual therapy, you probably garnered only a lukewarm response. After all, you've got presbyopia, which means "old eye." As your circulation slows down, the lenses of your eyes become dry and stiff, the muscles that control them weaken, and you can't focus up close anymore. It's a natural consequence of the aging process. Right?

Here's the popular theory: we still have cavemen's eyes. The average cave person didn't live beyond his or her teens. Around two hundred years ago we lived to about thirty-five. Even a hundred years ago, life expectancy wasn't much over forty. An individual had about a one-in-ten shot of seeing the age of sixty-five. Then—wham—technology evolved exponentially, and so did we. Eighty percent of Americans can now expect to live past sixty-five. In fact, barring disease, a healthy woman turning fifty today is likely to live into her nineties.

So what happens to a cave person's eyes? Not only do we far outlive the natural expiration date of our vision, our antiquated eyes were hardly designed to endure the environmental stresses of modern life. From sighting game across the prairie, it's a far cry to sitting under fluorescent lights and staring at a computer screen all day. Children are becoming nearsighted at earlier ages, and adults who had escaped that fate became presbyopic earlier with each passing year. Those ancient little organs of perception just can't be expected to cope. It's a wonder any of us can see at all!

But wait a minute. What's wrong with this picture? We're not just living longer lives, we're living *healthier* and longer lives. It's not only technology that's keeping us going, there's been a giant evolutionary leap. Our hearts, lungs, kidneys, and brains; every organ, function, and system is operating longer and longer at peak performance levels—except the eyes.

Except the eyes? How can this be? Have our primary sense organs, the eyes, which bring us 90 percent of our information about our world, been somehow accidentally left out of the evolution revolution? Why are they the only part of us not thriving while others do, in spite of environmental poisons and stress? I think that what we have here is the penultimate case of not being able to see the forest through the trees—"see" being the truly operative term. Our sense of sight is how we absorb information about our world, but it's also a barometer of our response to these inputs.

LITTLE CAMERAS, OR WINDOWS TO THE SOUL?

The standard explanation of our eyes as sophisticated little cameras has hung on because the structure of the eye was a good model for the camera. In both, entering light passes through a lens, which adjusts to focus it directly onto the surface where it's to be chemically recorded—the film of the camera or the retina of the eye. The similarities pretty much end here.

Granted, when anything goes wrong with the lens, the focusing mechanism of either the camera or the eye, a blurry image results. What goes wrong and how to fix it, however, are entirely different matters. Presbyopia, the inability to focus sharply for near vision, is a result of changes in the structure and function of your lenses. If they were as simple as the ones in cameras, you'd be able to pop into the drugstore and pick up a new pair whenever necessary.

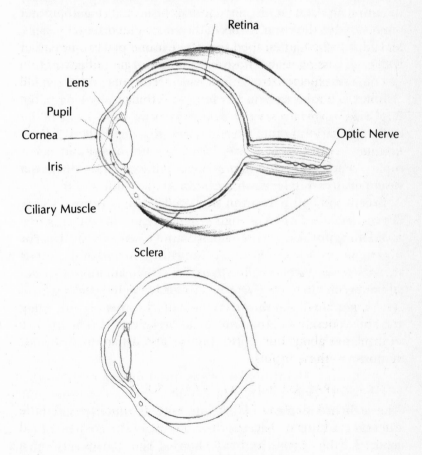

Illustration 1: The Human Eye

Scientists estimate that they now understand about 10 percent of the brain's workings and its potential. An identical figure applies to their knowledge of our visual system. This is because vision is a brain function; the eyes are literally extensions of the brain. During early gestation, the eyes are inside of the brain, and they gradually extend forward via a conduit of interconnected cells that become the optic nerves. At their tips are the brain cells that become the retina, the "film."

We don't see the images recorded on this film until they have passed down our optic nerves and been put together and interpreted by the visual cortex of the brain. This takes only a split second, but during that time an infinite number of reactions and responses take place that we are just beginning to understand.

The visual system and its little video recorders are incredibly complex. The average eye has nearly one billion working parts. A lot is going on in there! Dr. Robert-Michael Kaplan, one of the leading behavioral optometrists, notes in *Seeing Without Glasses* that our "eyes, for their size, have a greater blood and nerve supply than most other organ systems in the body, and there is a strong relationship between the brain and the fitness of the eyes. Approximately 49 percent of the brain's cranial nerves, which directly feed the body's nervous system, are just for the eyes." In addition, retinal nerve fibers make up 40 percent of all nerve fibers going to the brain. This is impressive in and of itself, but especially when you realize that the retina amounts to one-millionth of our body weight. Proportionately speaking, the eyes' requirements far outweigh those of our other organs. They are, for example, one-sixtieth of the weight of the heart, but their relative percentage of oxygen use is a full one-third of what the heart requires.

The brain is rightfully known as the three-pound universe, and the eyes are its galaxy of perception. Science can probe and dissect them till the end of time without discovering their innermost secrets. They're not measurably encoded in brain tissue, they belong in that realm beyond our instruments—the mind. It embodies our emotions and spirits, and influences are health and well-being—even our sight—in ways that science can rarely measure, much less control.

Our sight is essentially as individualistic as our thinking and feeling, and just as difficult to understand. In *Take Off Your*

Glasses and See, Dr. Jacob Liberman, another optometrist at the forefront of humanizing this science, puts it this way:

> Light energy enters our being through our eyes, but our vision of reality is determined more by what we see with our mind's eye than what we see with our physical eye. In fact, I found that our eyesight is simply a reflection of our view of reality. So when the mind begins to see more clearly, the eyes also begin to see more clearly...

This is looking less and less like a little book of eye exercises, isn't it?

HOW DO YOU FIX VISION?

Eye doctors Kaplan and Liberman broke from their traditional training when they realized that the conventional optometric approach not only doesn't cure most vision problems, it actually worsens many of them. Glasses can be compared to a cast on a broken leg. At first, they are a great artificial aid, but the longer they are used, the more the muscles atrophy and motor skills are lost.

The first eye doctor to make this connection and try to heal visual dysfunctions, instead of just compensate for them, was Dr. William H. Bates, a turn-of-the-century New York ophthalmologist. He declared that "mental tension" was at the root of all vision problems, and that sight could be naturally restored through relaxation and the retraining of visual skills and habits. However, instead of ushering in a revolutionary step in the world of vision, the Bates Method was soundly rejected by his scientific peers.

Both of the two main reasons for this rejection directly apply to presbyopia. Traditional optometric theory holds that the lens is entirely responsible for the process of accommodation, the shifting of focus on objects from distant to near. Bates's experiments led him to the conclusion, however, that it was the whole eye, rather than the lens, that changed shape to achieve this feat. It didn't matter that Bates's theory worked in practice, this sticking point over a technicality made him the black sheep of his profession.

Interestingly, today's debate is not over about what goes on during accommodation. The majority of research indicates that Bates's theory, which says that the whole eye and its extraocular muscles are involved, isn't correct. However, the accepted one, which states that the lens's shape changes through the pull of its attached ciliary muscles, also fails on occasion. Meanwhile, as arguments and studies continue, thousands of us are simply choosing to go with what works.

The Bates Method, upon which this program is based, works. Not just for nearsightedness and astigmatism, for which it's most famous, but for most other visual conditions, including presbyopia, that is, the inability to focus sharply for near vision. In fact, as Bates claims, "The first patient I cured of presbyopia was myself." A good reference, indeed. So, if this works, why doesn't every eye doctor practice it?

To flaunt convention in a conservative field is enough to get you ostracized, but the Bates Method and all its modern offshoots (including mine), also suffer from a spotty success record. Some people experience huge and lasting improvements, while others work hard for small and short-lived gains. Some days are clear, others are blurry. Inconsistencies like this can glaze over the eyes of a purely scientific mind. They're pretty frustrating for the rest of us too, but we take comfort in knowing that there are no cut-and-dried answers within the realm of the three-pound universe.

THE HOLISTIC VIEW

Even when individuals with reading glasses of the same strength prescription do exactly the same exercises for identical lengths of time, the results are liable to vary widely. Of the wide variety of factors accounting for this, some are physical and some are mental. The physical ones are fairly straightforward, while the mental ones are more complex.

On the physical level, the issue is primarily about getting increased circulation back into the eyes. Once they are again bathed in oxygen and nutrient-rich moisture, the lenses can soften up and regain their flexibility. There are prescribed exercises and massages to boost circulation, but the effects can be hampered by poor nutrition, lifestyle habits—as well as physical ones—and what Bates called "mental tension."

In the years since he used this phrase, our concepts of what constitutes mental tension have expanded about as much as our life span. It arises from a lot more than our specific problems and worries, or daily trials and tribulations. It's our reactions to these stresses that are the culprits, and these reactions are based on our expectations, beliefs, and attitudes toward ourselves, our vision, and life in general.

Since I began my career in the field of vision improvement because of my own nearsightedness, I quickly became aware of the emotional factors related to it. However, in true myopic fashion, I didn't pay much attention to any underlying emotional problems that might cause presbyopia until I experienced difficulty with my eyes. Even at fifty, I was surprised, because I had a healthy circulation and the added protection of some remaining mild myopia. Still, I couldn't help but notice that my arms seemed too short whenever I tried to read in poor lighting.

Naturally, I launched into my own personal presbyopia improvement program of exercises and nutrition. The timing just happened to coincide with my own personal mid-life crisis. Aging was on my mind—no wonder it was showing up in my eyes. Improving my visual skills would be no problem, but it was clearly time to get a better perspective on the whole situation.

A closer look revealed a great deal, some of it a little more than I was at first willing to see in myself. There's an enormous amount of subconscious conditioning behind the development and progression of presbyopia. In spite of twenty years of vision work, I'd fallen prey to some of it because I hadn't really understood how our beliefs about the aging process affect the course of this disease.

We are conditioned, you see, not to expect to be able to see clearly after a certain age. Failing eyesight afflicted our parents; we see virtually all "old" people with glasses, and eye doctors constantly remind us that it's coming. Pretty soon—what a surprise—our arms begin to shorten. We may fight it at first, but soon we resign ourselves to our fate. This fate is not just increasing poor eyesight, but the whole idea that aging and decline go hand in hand. As long as we hold on to this belief, no exercises or health regimen will have much effect.

Once we begin to experience deterioration of our vision, another kind of conditioning also begins to take hold. Each time we fail to see without glasses, we build to the expectation of future failures. This attitude is as detrimental to our vision as poor nutrition and bad circulation. On the whole, we get what we expect, so, again, exercises aren't very effective if they have an uphill battle against negative expectations.

I thought I had a perfect handle on positive expectations for vision and a good attitude about aging. However, the more I explored these attitudes, the more I found them to be a little shaky. Until I educated myself and "thought" my way out of them, they negated much of my vision work. As my ideas on aging shifted to truly positive views, my sight quickly cleared.

As I looked back on my presbyotic clients in the past, it was suddenly obvious that the ones who made the most progress had the best attitudes toward aging. Naturally, I began to incorporate exercises and information directly related to successful aging into my work with presbyopes. The results go far beyond improvements in vision and make my work more satisfying than ever before. Not only that, every time I help lift someone else's attitude, my own gets yet another boost. Lucky me!

THE TOTALLY TIMELESS TWENTY-EIGHT-DAY PROGRAM

Your attitudes on aging and your belief in your ability to see clearly again will have a definite impact on how much your vision will improve during the course of this program. So will your age, health, fitness, and the current strength of your glasses and how long you have worn them. Just as vital is your enjoyment factor. Boredom and drudgery aren't healing, but fun and adventure are salves to the body as well as the soul.

If you were in a workshop with me, you would definitely feel (and see) the spirit of fun and adventure playing its part. Under these circumstances, the best I can do is try to create that feeling in print. I'm going to pretend that this is a very long workshop that meets for a short time each morning. It's an unusual schedule, but we'll all work with it.

This program is all about flexibility! If you get bored, take a vacation for awhile. It doesn't matter if it takes you twenty-eight days or twenty-eight weeks to complete and integrate the material and exercises. The exercises are laid out in a gradual progression, but use them in any sequence you choose. You might want to read through the whole book before you begin the program. You will find lifestyle advice you might want to implement quickly, and any exercise that appeals to you can be put to use immediately.

What matters more to your eventual clarity is the spirit in which you enter each enterprise. Focus on it entirely. Find as much enjoyment in it as you can, and you'll get back far more than the time you put in. If you can't do an exercise or just don't like it, substitute something that's similar but more pleasurable, and you will get the benefits you need.

Each session of the program is broken into three sections: Attitude Adjustment, Lifestyle Adjustment, and Visual Adjustment. I call them adjustments because they ask for small rather than large changes. It is our natural tendency to resist huge shifts in our routines and thinking, but gradual ones will sink in and take effect.

Each of you taking part in this workshop has different eyes and different needs, and I've laid out something for everyone. To know what's right for you, trust your visual perception and your instincts, and don't worry about the rest. Let the concepts offered here bounce around in your brain, keep those ideas that appeal to you, and see what looks different in a month or so. I hope my ideas will be helpful, but nobody else has your vision.

THE PROGRAM

Let the workshop begin! Better yet, think of it as a "playshop." Improving your vision will take time and effort, but approaching the task in a spirit of fun and adventure is the secret weapon that will bring you the greatest success as well as the pleasure of enjoyment.

The attitude, lifestyle, and visual adjustments for each day this week are designed to prime your eyes, mind, and body to work together in the re-creation of your near-point clarity. Still, many of you will notice encouraging progress right away if you haven't been wearing glasses too long and are in reasonably good physical condition. Be patient, and always expect the best!

Be especially patient with the process of harnessing your mental powers during the Breathing Affirmation section of Attitude Adjustment. If you've had no practice with mental techniques such as meditation or self-hypnosis, you may have some initial difficulty maintaining your concentration. Besides exercising patience, you may also find it helpful to enlist the aid of a tape recorder, a friend, or both. Having the directions read to you, live or on tape, can greatly ease the process. In fact, you may want to record the instructions to any exercise you have trouble remembering. Better yet, do the whole program with a partner.

Patient persistence is also the key to establishing a new habit this week! Be open to the possibility of seeing clearly whenever you pick up something to read. I can't even begin to estimate how many times I've caught people using their glasses when they don't actually need them. Always give your eyes a chance to function on their own before you resort to artificial assistance. They may happily surprise you!

Here's what you'll need besides this book:

MATERIALS LIST

1. A pair of reading glasses one-half diopter weaker than your current prescription. You will probably go through a series of them as you work your way through the program. The inexpensive ones from the drugstore are generally okay. However, the low-quality glass can cause distortions which bring on eyestrain. If your eyes tire or burn, or you get headaches, look into a higher quality pair of glasses.
2. Photocopies of:
The Bookmark (page 14)

The Mandala Stretch—week two (page 99)
Near and Far Charts—week two (page 107)
The Spiral—week three (page 127)
The Mazes—week three (page 144)
The Labyrinth—week four (page 190)
Number Bounce—week four (page 197)

3. Fusion String—week two. A three-foot length of string with knots tied in it every two inches. A bright color is best. The nylon line used in construction is excellent.

4. A big ball or minitrampoline—week two. You can get by without one, but they are highly recommended, especially the ball. I am referring to those huge spheres used for exercising. They range in size from twenty-five inches to thirty-six inches in diameter. You will want one small enough so that you can sit on it comfortably, but big enough so that your knees are not above the level of your thighs. These balls are one of the great inventions of our time. They're wonderful as furniture. Get one!

5. Music. Also optional but highly recommended. Music will help with the relaxation, concentration, and movement that will contribute to your better vision. Rhythmic instrumental selections are best. Some of the best choices are:
Pachelbel's Canon in D
Mozart's Piano Concerto no. 21 ("Elvira Madigan")
Strauss waltzes
Chariots of Fire by Vangelis
Brahms's "lullaby"
Your favorite music

THE BOOKMARK

To make this a lasting, effective tool, xerox the bookmark on the following page (why not try using bright-colored paper!), and have it laminated at a copy shop. To use: Place the bookmark two pages ahead of you whenever you read anything, including this book. When you reach the marker, follow its instructions, and place it ahead two more pages (and so on).

BOOKMARK

- Take off your glasses!

- Yawn—at least 3 times.

- Stand up and stretch (or stretch while sitting).

- Stretch your eye muscles: look up, down, left, right, diagonally, and around in circles.

- Shift your focus quickly, in and out 5 times, from near to distant objects.

- Palm for at least 5 deep breaths.

- Put the bookmark ahead 2 pages and continue reading, first checking to see if you can read without your glasses.

PART ONE

THE PROGRAM

DAY ONE

Because the mind influences every cell in the body, human aging is fluid and changeable; it can speed up, slow down, stop for a time, and even reverse itself.

Deepak Chopra, M.D.
Ageless Body, Timeless Mind

ATTITUDE ADJUSTMENT

Until 1983, I had a tough time convincing skeptics that our power of vision is a fluid, ever-changing process capable of growth and expansion rather than a mechanical function doomed to continual deterioration. No matter how many inspirational anecdotal case studies I related, they stubbornly insisted on the need for "scientific proof." I would patiently explain that the role of the mind in vision made pure research difficult, but the hard-core skeptics still weren't impressed.

Finally, in 1983, a research study turned up. This was not just any old study, but one that would more than satisfy the doubters. It proved that vision could change to an absolutely mind-boggling degree. My job suddenly was a lot easier.

This study took place in Chicago, and has been duplicated in a number of later research projects. In each, psychiatrists working with patients suffering from multiple personality disorder had their clients examined by eye doctors. As the therapists guided the patients through a process of shifting from one personality to another, the eye doctors ran their battery of tests. I wish I could have seen their expressions.

The psychiatrists had already observed that the separate personalities of their patients often wore different prescription glasses. One persona might be a fifteen-year-old myope (near-sighted), another a middle-aged presbyope (far-sighted). The researcher's question: Was the visual change organic, or was it a hallucinatory manifestation of the mental illness? The answer: real physical changes occurred.

The machines measured significant alterations in acuity, refraction, and the actual shape and curvature of the eyes. Nearsightedness, farsightedness, astigmatism—all moved flu-idly from one persona to the next. One woman who suffered from multiple personality disorder even had amblyopia—"lazy eye blindness," in which the nerves of one eye shut down—in one personality but not her other two. Cataracts and glaucoma came and went. The case considered most astounding was a man who was color-blind, which is considered genetically unalterable, in one personality but not others. Ah, the mysteries of the three-pound universe!

So there you have it, the same physical body can house the eyes in different personalities, including those of both a young and an old person. As the quotation which began this section points out, not only can the aging process speed up, slow down, stop for a time, and even reverse itself, it can even do so virtually instantaneously.

Aging and vision are fluid and flexible. We don't have to be mentally ill to act on this reality. All we have to do is believe in it and go after it. You'll read about some of my clients who have done just that, but I also urge you to delve into this topic more extensively on your own. Deepak Chopra's *Ageless Body, Timeless Mind* is a great place to start. The more you boost your belief in your regenerative potential, the more clearly you'll literally see it happen.

Of course, this is generally easier said than done. Even if we already consciously and intellectually believe in this potential, we still have an uphill battle against our early subconscious conditioning. To counter this, we need all the positive recondi-tioning we can get.

That's why the Attitude Adjustment exercise for today and every day of the program is so important. I call it the Breathing

Affirmation. While in a state of relaxation, you'll be mentally repeating all or part of the quotation for the day in time with your breathing. This simple and pleasant procedure, which you can call self-hypnosis or meditation or any of the many mental focusing techniques, is designed to bring your intellectual understanding down into your subconscious belief system, where you can truly internalize it. And it takes less than five minutes.

These minutes will most likely be even more pleasant and productive if you use background music. Whatever you find the most soothing and relaxing is perfect for right now, while something more rhythmic and upbeat will be best for the physical and vision exercises.

BREATHING AFFIRMATION

For this exercise, you can either sit or lie down. Be comfortable, but don't cross your arms or legs. Your eyes will be closed throughout.

There are three steps to this process: accessing your sub-conscious by relaxing as deeply as possible, mentally repeating the affirmation in time with your breathing, and then bringing yourself back to full alertness.

Step One: Focus your attention on taking ten slow deep breaths. Use your imagination and think how breathing would feel if you were a balloon. As you gradually fill up with air, experience it as a sensation of gentle stretching and expansion throughout your entire body, like you're a balloon blowing up. As you let each breath out, imagine you are going limp and relaxed, just like a balloon with the air leaking out of it.

Mentally count each exhalation, from ten down to one. Think "ten" on your first breath out, "nine" on the second, and so on. You may feel a sensation of sinking downward with each descending number. This is good. Enjoy it. You're going deeper down inside yourself.

After you have breathed and relaxed your way down to "one," enjoy the pleasant feelings of relaxation for a few more breaths.

Step Two: Switch over to synchronizing your breathing with

the affirmation, while continuing to experience the sensation of your whole body breathing.

The affirmation for today is: "Aging can slow down and reverse itself."

As you inhale, think: "Aging can slow down."

As you exhale, think: "And reverse itself."

Do this for ten breaths (longer if you like).

Step Three: When you are finished, luxuriate in the feelings of well-being for a few moments. Then bring yourself back to full alertness by taking three deep breaths, each fuller and more energetic than the one before. Count up mentally but enthusiastically on your inhalations: One, two, three! Finish by opening your eyes and thinking, or saying out loud, "Wide awake and refreshed!" Enjoy a stretch and yawn!

How do you feel? Was this a simple matter for you or a challenge to your concentration and imagination? Some of us are naturals at focusing our attention and going inside, but it's a learned skill for the majority of us. If it wasn't easy for you, stick with it—the benefits are worth the effort.

LIFESTYLE ADJUSTMENT

Although the mind may greatly influence both vision and the aging process, the better the material it has to work with, the easier the job will be. Every now and then someone amazes me by achieving significant and lasting visual improvement in spite of an unhealthy lifestyle, but those rare souls are few and far between. The rest of us have to make some effort to get more oxygen-filled, nutrient-rich circulation into our eyes.

Only you can decide how much of what is offered in this program is a necessary addition to your current lifestyle. However, even if you're already very physically active, there's a good chance you're still not getting circulation all the way up into your eyes.

If you already practice yoga, you're on the right track. Stretching, inversion, and breathing bring up the regenerating supercirculation our eyes and brain need as we age. We'll be using other approaches as well, such as massage and nutrition, but we'll start off right now with some easy movement and breathing exercises that will produce big results.

One note of caution before we begin: if you have any medical conditions, especially high blood pressure or glaucoma, be sure to check with your physician before doing any of the physical exercises, especially those that involve inversion. That said, let me stress that while everything presented here is gentle, you are on your honor to progress at a pace that is comfortable for you. Forget about "more pain, more gain." It's an unnatural and counterproductive philosophy. In truth, less pain brings more gain. We shrink from pain and grow from pleasure. Your goal is to feel good!

Don't be surprised if you have a burst of clearer vision after this first session. So check out how your vision is now. Take your glasses off and observe the degree of blurriness of the print. Notice how far away you're holding the book.

Of course, keep your glasses off as you do the exercises, but let your music go right on playing—it'll enhance grace and ease of movement. Enjoy!

Before you start this circulation-boosting, wake-up routine of Stretching and Curling [illustrations 2a, 2b, and 2c], close your eyes for a few moments and notice how you feel now. Take a survey of your eyes, face, breathing, back, legs, and general state of well-being.

Inhale deeply and stretch up, feeling the stretch from your fingers to your toes. Move your stretch from side to side by lifting the heel opposite the side that you're stretching higher.

Stretch this way for at least two or three minutes, and as you do *yawn!* The whole time! Big noisy yawns! Express yourself! *This is an order: Do not skimp on your yawns!* You are flooding your eyes with massive doses of circulation. You can feel it as an increase in moisture.

Ah, there. Good. Relax.

Now let's use inversion and loosen your spine while the circulation goes deeper into your whole visual system.

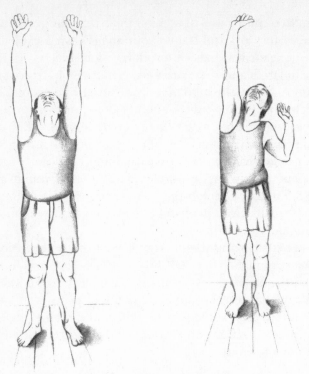

Illustration 2a and b: Stretching

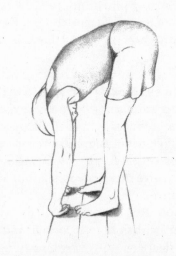

Illustration 2c: Curling

First, take in a deep inhalation. Start exhaling as you relax your head forward and down. Continue this long exhalation as your head leads your spine toward your feet. Keep your knees a little bent, arms and shoulders relaxed. Look back through your legs rather than at the floor in front of your feet, so that your neck remains relaxed.

When you're hanging all the way over, take in another deep inhalation.

Exhale gradually as you curl your way back up. Keep your knees bent, tuck your hips under, and feel how your vertebrae are stacking as you straighten.

When you're completely erect, inhale; exhale as you curl down again, and so on.

Do this at least six times (unless, as with anything else, you feel discomfort).

Finally, close your eyes, survey yourself again, and compare how you feel now to how you felt before you began.

Take another look at this page without your glasses. If there's not at least a brief improvement, rest assured that it will come with more time and practice.

How did your spine respond to the stretching and loosening? A very true yoga saying reminds us, "You are as young as your spine is supple." Thus, you've just taken a step into age reversal! Can you feel it yet?

VISUAL ADJUSTMENT

Long Swings [illustration 3] increase circulation, limber the spine, and restore the natural vibratory movement of the eyes. Our heartbeats are matched by a corresponding "beat" by our eyes, which is really a vibration, because it is more like seventy to eighty beats per second than per minute. When tension and slow circulation enter the picture, there is less movement in the eyes, and they lose some of their ability to rapidly scan for and record details.

This is another important time for music. The longer you stay with and enjoy the rhythmic movement of Long Swings, the more you will gain from them. Swinging is a very pleasurable sensation, but it's so simple and repetitive that many people are quickly bored by it. With the addition of music, however, interest is held by the rhythm and mood evoked.

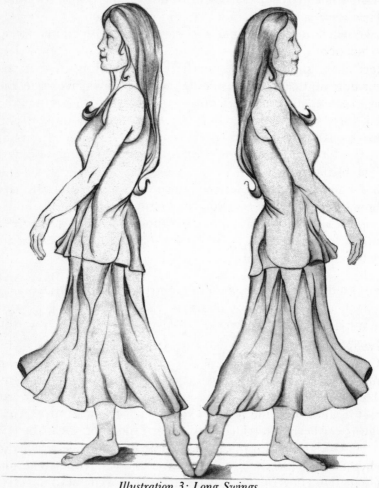

Illustration 3: Long Swings

For example, swinging to Brahms's "lullaby" can bring up feelings of loving tenderness not only toward your eyes, but also toward your whole self and others. Another good choice is

Mozart's Piano Concerto no. 21, popularly known as the Theme
From Elvira Madigan. To garner a sense of freshness and
exhilaration, move in time to Pachelbel's *Canon*. Feel in the need
of personal strength? Swing to Vangelis's *Chariots of Fire*. Just
want to feel light and happy? Try any of the Strauss waltzes.
How about a sensuous experience? Ravel's *Bolero* will definitely
take you to new realms of physical pleasure!

Stand as shown in the illustration, evenly balanced with your
feet about shoulder-width apart. You are merely going to be
turning your body from side to side. When you rotate to the
right, your left heel comes off the ground. As you swing to the
left, your right heel will come up. Let your arms simply hang
like loose ropes. They should stay so relaxed that at the end of
each turn they flop against your body.

Keep your eyes aligned with the movement of your head and
body. Don't focus on anything, just let the view slide by. You may
notice that as you swing in one direction the view slides by in the
opposite direction. This illusion of motion is something that you
will be working with a lot in the upcoming days and weeks.

After you have been swinging for only a minute, you can
actually feel the life and vibration coming back to your eyes.
This is not part of the actual exercise, just something to do once
so you really know what is happening.

Try this self-demonstration: Close one eye as you keep on
swinging, and *very gently* touch your closed lid with a fingertip.
Can you feel your eye vibrating? If your eyes have been tense, it
may even feel like they're jerking or leaping around in there.
That's the natural vibration as it starts up again. However you
feel it, know that the movement is good. Then, let your hand
down slowly, and keep on swinging.

As you swing, keep your mind clear; lose yourself in the
rhythm and mood of the music. Breathe easily, but deeply. On
every fourth exhalation or so, blink softly but rapidly for its
duration. Swing for at least three minutes.

When you're finished, notice how calmly energized you and
your eyes feel. Can you feel energy streaming down your arms

and through your hands? You may also feel a lightness in your arms and hands, as if they want to float up. Enjoy it—it's merely a fun side effect from an exercise that benefits your entire body.

Today, and every day during the program, let what you've learned and accomplished seep into your thoughts and activities. There's no requirement to put in a certain amount of time, but whenever you are consciously aware of your vision and connecting with it, you are developing it. Consider the following list of suggestions, and see if you can seize brief opportunities to do something good for your vision and entire being.

TODAY

- Let the phrase "aging can slow down, stop, and reverse itself" play through your mind.
- Start using this week's bookmark.
- Yawn a lot.
- Refresh yourself a few times with some stretching and curling up and down.
- Loosen your eyes with several minutes of Long Swings.
- Before reading, check to see if you can use your weaker glasses or none at all.
- Read tomorrow's material before going to bed tonight.

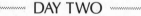

DAY TWO

You'll see it when you believe it.

Dr. Wayne Dyer

ATTITUDE ADJUSTMENT

I love the way Wayne Dyer turned the old axiom, I'll believe it when I see it, into the title of his inspirational book, *You'll See It When You Believe It.* This is a truism for life in general. A healthy skepticism is a valuable tool in certain circumstances, but by and large we get what we believe. I see this belief validated all the time in the course of my work.

It's been a good many years now, but the first time I encountered an obvious display of the power of belief on vision still sticks in my mind. The client, Betty, just happened to be a presbyope. (That's what you're called when you have pres-byopia, and it's sometimes affectionately shortened to "presby.") She was one of my very first vision students, a forty-eight-year-old homemaker who came to me because she hated, and kept losing or breaking, the reading glasses she had needed for the past four years.

Betty was a sweet woman who never had a bad thing to say about anyone, with the glaring exception of herself. She constantly described herself as inept, and was one of those people who apologizes for things not even remotely her fault.

Every time she experienced a clear view of a printed page she would exclaim, "I can't believe I can see this!" And, every time, poof!, her clarity would vanish. Even though my experience was limited and my understanding of the power of belief only at an instinctual level, I knew I was right in saying that her response was the cause of her vanishing clarity. We went over this constantly, but self-doubt was ingrained in Betty's identity. After two months of conscientious practice, her ability to read without glasses was still minimal. We had to settle for some skills that would help her out when her glasses were lost or broken.

Twenty years ago, I emphasized the importance of affirmations to Betty and other clients. I knew this belief system had to be enlisted in the visual healing and reeducation process. I just didn't know what it really took to accomplish this feat. Simple affirmations for positive change and beliefs have all the right stuff in them, but to get results by repeating them at the left-brain, analytical, conscious level takes an awfully long time. To really take hold, the messages have to get all the way down to the subconscious portion of the brain.

The quickest and most successful way to accomplish this is by using mental techniques which combine deep relaxation, imagination, and focused concentration. I came to understand this phenomenon about ten years ago when I was training to become a hypnotherapist. I had been drawn to the training after reading numerous articles about hypnosis and healing. When I applied what I learned to my own vision work, my acuity jumped and I was able to keep it with far less effort than before. My clients had similar results. I found myself putting this expanded approach into book form for the general public, which became *Hypnovision: The New Natural Way to Vision Improvement*. This was the second book I'd written about vision improvement. The first was *Visionetics: The Holistic Way to Better Eyesight*. In those early years, I knew that the people who improved the most were those who did the exercises in what I could only describe then as a "deeply meditative state of mind." With the simple tools provided by hypnosis, I was finally better able to help more people across this mental province where miracles can take place.

What you have here as your Breathing Affirmations are self-hypnosis exercises similar to the ones in *HypnoVision*. If you felt relaxed and could even vaguely experience the idea of your body breathing, you "hypnotized" yourself during the first such exercise, yesterday. It's not any sort of strange or mystical state, it's just relaxing into your subconscious mode of thinking. Hypnosis differs from techniques going by such names as meditation, creative visualization, and progressive relaxation only in that it is more specifically goal-orientated, more con-sciously directed at changing subconscious programming.

Over the years, I've lost contact with Betty, but I've often wished I could go back in time. It would be a joy to teach her this technique for reestablishing her belief in herself and her vision. I suspect she would be a little fearful and resistant at first. The word *hypnosis* might carry negative connotations for her. I'd turn that around for her, though, by explaining that, in essence, she is already hypnotized: She is conditioned at the subconscious level with negative beliefs and expectations. Therefore, what we are really going to do is "dehypnotize" her to get rid of the misconceptions that obscure the truth.

If you've had any lingering doubts about hypnosis, I hope this explanation will also satisfy you. Let Betty's story remind you to stick with and continue to develop your skills with the Attitude Adjustment sections of the program. Remember, even if you already consciously believe the affirmations, your subconscious has been influenced by all those years of being told that reading glasses come with aging. Don't keep sabotaging your own best efforts by underestimating the power of suggestion, whether it's positive or negative.

So, as you do today's Breathing Affirmation, start exploring and developing your ability to enter this perfectly natural and extremely pleasurable state of mind. You'll be aware of everything going on around you, but your aim is to be in your own private world at the same time. Let outside sounds and any extraneous thoughts float by. Relax, use your imagination, feel your breathing, and enjoy the soothing reassurance of the affirmations.

BREATHING AFFIRMATION

Settle down into a comfortable position, close your eyes, and begin relaxing. Enjoy being still and taking this time to go within. Focus on your breathing. Let it be easy and deep, like your whole body is breathing, and count these breaths from ten down to one.

Savor the deep relaxation.

For another ten or more slow breaths, mentally repeat the following affirmation:

Inhaling: "I believe."

Exhaling: "My vision is regenerating."

After ten repetitions, relax for a few more breaths with the satisfied feeling that the affirmation has brought.

Then, breathe and count up from one to three, reminding yourself that you're wide awake and refreshed.

LIFESTYLE ADJUSTMENT

While you were doing your Breathing Affirmation, your eyes were getting an extra bonus. The physical relaxation and breathing brought an added dose of circulation into your eyes.

Now we'll open it more, first with a variation of stretching and curling, and then with a new breathing technique. Remember to adapt the directions to your own personal readiness. Stay comfortable!

Begin by closing your eyes and becoming aware of how you feel now—eyes, whole body, and mood.

Begin yawning and stretching up. Luxuriate in this for at least ten long yawns. Relax and enjoy the results.

Move on to exhaling as you curl forward and down, remembering to keep your knees slightly bent and to look back through your legs, rather than in front of your feet.

While you're hanging over, loosen up your legs and back a bit by flopping gently from side to side. Let your movement be so soft that it's not quite a bounce. Flop back and forth at least six times, breathing easily and deeply.

Now, let's loosen up your neck muscles while you're still hanging over.

Keep breathing deeply as you let your head gently swing back and forth, from side to side, about a dozen times. Don't lift it, just let it swing easily. Notice that you can feel the muscles on each side of your neck being softly stretched.

Curl back up and exhale.

Continue with the basic pattern, but changing the direction of your head swings each time you hang over.

The next one is a front-to-back swing, then diagonally up right and down left, and finally, up left and down right.

Do complete circles of your head around to the right.

Then, do complete circles of your head around to the left.

When you are finished, be aware of how you feel.

Can you feel the warmth of circulation in your neck? How are your face, back, eyes, and even your mood? How's your vision? Without your glasses, take a look at this page. Is there an immediate effect?

Next, it's time to spend just a few minutes with a breathing "exercise" that will be the basis for all your breathing during this program and can transform your entire sense of well-being. I say "exercise" because Abdominal Breathing [illustration 4] is really our natural way of breathing. In a few days we'll delve more fully into this topic, but suffice it to say now that breathing only with your chest vastly reduces your intake of oxygen.

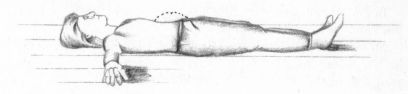

Illustration 4: Abdominal Breathing

You can, of course, breathe this way sitting or standing, but lying down is a relaxing way to practice. If your lower back is not comfortable with your legs straight, it's fine to bend your knees or put a pillow under them.

Start by tightening your abdominal muscles as you exhale completely.

Relax these muscles as you inhale, letting your belly expand like a balloon.

Exhale gradually, using your abdominal muscles.

That's all there is to it. (It may seem strange at first if you've been used to pulling these muscles in with your breaths in, but stick with it and you'll soon be a pro at what nature intended.)

Keep practicing for at least ten breaths.

Ah, isn't that pleasant and relaxing? You get to do more now, because this breath is also part of today's Visual Adjustment.

VISUAL ADJUSTMENT

How's your vision right now without glasses? After you've checked it and read the directions, keep your glasses off during the exercises.

Put on the music you used yesterday for swinging, or try another selection. You'll want to leave it on once we move from the swings into a new exercise.

Begin your Long Swings, but do them with your eyes closed for the first minute or so. Focus on feeling your eyes loosening up and beginning to vibrate freely.

Then open your eyes for the duration of your swinging to the music. Let your gaze slide right over the view you're swinging by. Breathe deeply and regularly, and every now and then blink quickly and softly during an exhalation.

Take a peek at the printed page when you're finished.

Now it's time for the Lens Flexor [illustration 5], a remarkable mind-and-body exercise. You'll be stimulating the flexibility of your lenses through a synchronized combination of imagination, hand movement, and breathing. You'll actually be able to feel the sensation in your eyes!

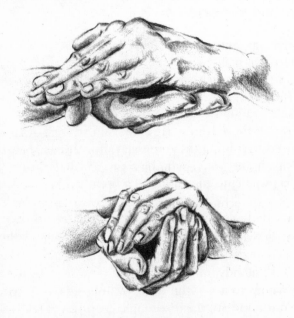

Illustration 5: The Lens Factor

Sit comfortably with both feet flat on the floor. Hold your hands as you see in the illustration, as if you were holding something delicate cupped between them. The hand movement you will make will be soft and simple. Just alternate back and forth between the round cupped position and one in which your hands flatten out so your palms become parallel to each other, about one inch apart.

Breathe through your nose, synchronized with the movement of your hands. Inhale as you "round" your hands; exhale as you flatten them. Let your breaths be easy, but make each one full. Let your stomach also round out as you inhale. Tighten your abdominal muscles as you exhale and flatten your hands.

Keep your eyes *closed* throughout. Be aware that your hands are moving in the same way you desire your lenses to flex and change shape. Add the power of your mind to your movement and breathing. Imagine you can feel this same movement in the lenses of your eyes. This takes less imagination than you might think. You should feel the sensation of movement almost immediately.

Stay with this exercise for at least two minutes.

Isn't that an amazing sensation? Can you feel that your lenses have had a little work out? You've loosened them up and increased circulation to them in a variety of ways today. How does this page look to your lens-free vision?

TODAY

- Let the affirmation, "I believe my vision is regenerating," play through your thoughts.
- Use the Lens Flexor exercise several times—even fifteen or twenty seconds of it will loosen your lenses and open your breathing.
- Relax your spine and neck at least once by curling over and swinging your head.
- Take a body, mind, and vision minivacation by doing Long Swings to a favorite piece of music.
- Yawn and stretch as often as possible, sitting or standing.
- Read tomorrow's material tonight.

DAY THREE

Belief creates biology.

Norman Cousins

ATTITUDE ADJUSTMENT

This morning let's dwell a little more on the impact of the mind on both healing and quality of life. No doubt you have heard of a phenomenon called the placebo effect. It is the most amazing and potentially powerful agent in the healing process, yet it is generally regarded by science as something which just interferes with research. Built into nearly every medical study is a percentage of responses that must be discounted due to the placebo effect. In essence, it is a healing response triggered on by the individual's belief that the medical procedure or drug will work.

There are countless examples of the placebo effect in action. Let me offer one here that ties in with another condition that generally comes in conjunction with aging: angina pectoris, the frightening and often debilitating heart pain that crops up when coronary arteries are blocked. When a minor surgical procedure developed during the 1950s had exciting results, a controlled study was then done to rule out the placebo effect. To the great consternation of the innovative surgical team, there was an equal amount of heart muscle function improvement in the group of men who thought they were having the full surgery when, in fact, they were merely incised and then sewn back up. Belief creates biology.

When our minds are truly engaged in reversing the aging process, we also get what we believe. The nature of your thoughts will influence your vision as well as every other aspect of your mental and physical health. I see this in my clients, and research backs it up.

For example, in the late 1970s, a Harvard team led by psychologist Ellen Langer showed that vision was one of a myriad of age indicators that can rejuvenate with the kind of mental shifts I call attitude adjustments. The study isolated a group of men in their seventies in a time warp. They lived for a week in an environment carefully constructed to duplicate their lives when they were in their fifties. Their job was to *believe* they were living twenty years ago.

The results were astounding. By the end of the week there was a significant measurable change in the senses of vision, hearing, taste, as well as manual dexterity, physical strength, short-term memory, and other indicators of biological age. And how about this: there was in increase in finger length. Our fingers shorten as we grow older, but in one week these men had actually regenerated the fingers of younger bodies. Wow!

There are three types of age: chronological, psychological, and biological. We can't change chronology, but the rest is fluid; and our psychological age heavily influences our biological age. To paraphrase Henry Ford, whether you think of yourself as young or old, you're right.

BREATHING AFFIRMATION

Feel your whole body breathe as you count down from ten to one. Pause to enjoy. For your next ten slow breaths:

Inhale: "I am creating."

Exhale: "younger vision."

Luxuriate in the effects. Breathe and count up from one to three, and say "Alert and refreshed!"

I see belief creating biology all the time in my work. A few years after the not-so-happy story of Betty who couldn't believe, I worked with another Betty. This one was a fifty-five-year-old myope, a people-shy but nature-loving watercolor artist. However, she rarely wore her distance glasses and had no interest in changing her nearsightedness. Betty loved seeing and painting the world in a Monet-like softness, but now her near vision was starting to blur too. Painting the far-off blur was one thing, having the paint itself blur was quite another.

Even though Betty was a shy introvert, she was comfortable with herself and confident in her talents. She was also a lifelong

Christian Scientist and had an absolute belief in natural healing. Her personal program relied as heavily on the healing power of prayer, enlisting the aid of her church's practitioners, as it did on the vision exercises. Within a week, she was seeing her paints clearly again.

LIFESTYLE ADJUSTMENT

Before we go on, how about enjoying a few Stretches, yawns, and Curls? While you're hanging over from the waist, be sure to spend a little time loosening your neck.

There, that's better. How do your eyes see and feel?

In the Harvard study of the men who reversed the aging process, one of the happy results was that the men's faces looked three to five years younger after the experiment. This is an effect you can also expect as you rejuvenate your eyesight, especially as you incorporate today's exercise into your lifestyle. It's simply called the Facial Massage [illustration 6]. You'll be invigorating as well as relaxing your face, and circulation and energy will also flood into your eyes. Playing beautiful background music can enhance the effects.

Before you begin, take a good look at your face in a mirror. Your warm-up stretches have already brought circulation into your face, but the Facial Massage will bring up a lot more.

Close your eyes (and keep them closed) and focus your attention on what sensations, or lack of them, you feel throughout your face as well as in and around your eyes.

Now, begin with your eyebrows. Take an eyebrow between the thumb and first finger of each hand, and knead and squeeze your way back and forth across them. Be firm, but don't cause yourself great pain. (The tenderness will dissipate with continued practice.) Close your eyes as you massage, and keep this up for at least four deep abdominal breaths.

Next, move on to your forehead. Use the fingers of both hands and massage all over your forehead, paying special attention to your temples and the space above and between your eyebrows.

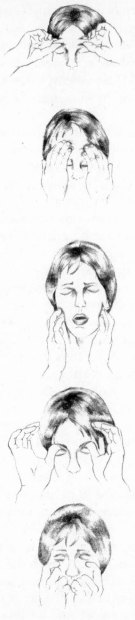

Illustration 6: Facial Massage

You want this to feel firmly invigorating as well as loosening, but be a little more gentle on your temples. Keep your attention on the sensation and do this for at least four long breaths.

Now locate your jaw muscles (you may have to open and close your mouth to do this). Take at least three more breaths as you massage away their tension. This is also a good time for a few extra yawns.

Moving on from your jaw muscles, give the rest of your face a gentle going over. Pay special attention to the area above your upper lip.

Then, avoid your eyelids, but let your fingers lightly tap and dance all over your face. And yawn!

Finally, concentrate on the bones around your eyes. Without putting any pressure on your eyes themselves, use your thumbs along the top ridge of bone, and your first fingers along the bottom ridge. Don't forget the outer corners where the upper and lower areas come together—these are important ac-cupressure points. In fact, so are any other sensitive areas you locate along these bones. They are also related to sinus function-ing, so you are getting a little something extra. Breathe deeply as you massage the area three or four times.

When you're finished, keep your eyes closed for a few moments and enjoy the vitality you feel in your face and eyes.

Can you read any more clearly without glasses? Go back to your mirror and see how much age reversal you've accomplished!

VISUAL ADJUSTMENT

Now we're going to take the concept of age reversal to really grand heights. First, however, put on a piece of rhythmic music for a round of Long Swings with an added variation.

Extend the index finger of your right hand up and directly out in front of you at arm's length, with the nail towards you at eye level. Notice how clearly you can now see the details of this fingernail. If you can see it clearly, move it in toward you until the image begins to blur.

As you swing, keep your focus on your fingernail, which

moves right along with your body and eyes. Be aware that the background is zooming past you in the opposite direction of your swing. This stimulates even more movement and circulation in your eyes.

Breathe and blink!

After several minutes, change hands and keep on swinging.

Finally, stop, relax, and notice how you feel and see.

Our new exercise for today will have a physical effect on your eyes, but it's really about aiming your mental power directly at the age-reversal process for your vision.

One of the first rules of hypnosis is to give suggestions for the most positive possible outcome. Give the mind the highest goal to shoot for and it will achieve more than if you give it a more moderate, or "realistic," target. In our case, the most complete age reversal imaginable would be to the eyes of a baby.

Imagination is the key word here. Research in the field of healing through imagery has consistently found that the more vividly the image is seen or emotionally felt, the greater the positive results. It has been found, too, that the emotion which precipitates the deepest healing is love.

So, today's vision exercise is really an introduction to your eyes from a while new perspective. Regarded as inanimate machines, they'll continue to fail you. Treated as integral and beloved parts of your whole being, they'll regenerate and remain healthy and vital.

Your job here is to become actively involved in anthropomorphizing your eyes, in giving them character and personality. Until now they've been old codgers, neglected and tired, undernourished and let to atrophy. So, poof! Let's transform them into a pair of newborn twins.

I call this Rocking the Babies. You may find taping these instructions very helpful for your emotional involvement. If you can't get into the mood, just relax and enjoy the swaying movement that will loosen your eyes and flood them with circulation. On the other hand, you may find this a moving experience. When I do this with groups there is no shortage of beaming expressions of love, tears, and even arms held up as if truly cradling and rocking a cherished baby.

This is also a prime time to use rhythmic, evocative music, especially a lullaby or romantic piece. Brahms's "lullaby" is an excellent choice, but go with a personal favorite if you have one. Mine, for example, is "Little Buckaroo," a very old Bing Crosby song which my father cowrote. I sing it as I rock, just as my father did to me, and it never fails to evoke loving feelings. Perhaps there's one you used to soothe a baby, and you can now hum or sing it to yourself.

Sit in a comfortable chair that allows you room to move a little from side to side. Close your eyes and bring your attention to them.

Let your torso sway from left to right in time with the music as you shift your weight from one hip to the other.

Sense your eyes floating gently from side to side.

Think of them as babies. You may have a visual image of them, or just the idea and feeling.

These babies had become weak and atrophied from lack of attention and nourishment, but they are responding to your care and attention. They float from side to side, relaxing, becoming infused with health and energy.

As you lovingly rock these babies, the muscles in and around your eyes are relaxing. Circulation is opening and flowing freely into them. They are becoming healthier and younger.

Continue to rock them for three to five minutes.

Then, before opening your eyes, spend a few moments noticing how they feel.

What was your experience? How did you feel emotionally? It's not uncommon to have a brief leap in visual acuity after this exercise. Can you read any more clearly without your glasses?

TODAY

- Own the thought, "I am creating younger vision."
- Yawn and stretch as often as possible.

- Curl your spine up and down a few times.
- When you rest your eyes from reading, breathe abdominally and use the Lens Flexor.
- Do a few Long Swings whenever there's a beautiful view to let slide by in the other direction.
- Refresh your face and eyes with a Facial Massage.
- Read tomorrow's material.

DAY FOUR

He lives most life whoever breathes the most air.

Elizabeth Barrett Browning

Breathing is the key that unlocks the whole catalog of advanced biological function and development. Is it any wonder that it is so central to every aspect of health?

Sheldon Saul Hendler, M.D.
The Oxygen Breakthrough

Breathing in, I calm body and mind.
Breathing out I smile.
Dwelling in this present moment,
I know this is the only moment.

Thich Nhat Hanh

ATTITUDE ADJUSTMENT

Three quotations about breathing? Yes. After all, if you're alive you must be breathing, right? Yes and no. Minimal breathing will keep you on this plane of existence, but it takes *real* breathing to feel fully alive. If by some bizarre twist of fate I had to limit myself to teaching only one thing, it wouldn't be vision improvement, yoga, or self-hypnosis. It would be breathing.

In yoga, the word closest to *air* is *prana*, which translates literally as "life force." *Spiritus* is the Latin word for "breath." In Hebrew, God is called Yahweh, which also means "wind." Poets, spiritual leaders, philosophers, yogis, psychologists, and doctors know of the powers and mysteries that lie within our breath.

Breathing is our most fundamental key to health, well-being, and even spiritual connection. You've already heard me repeat its necessity in vision work over and over. Yet I know from experience that this is a message people often have difficulty grasping and integrating. It calls for an attitude adjustment.

Our modern world has produced nothing less than an epidemic of oxygen deprivation. The full title of Dr. Hendler's revealing book is *The Oxygen Breakthrough: 30 Days to an Illness-Free Life*. He is just one of a growing number of medical doctors who now realize the far-reaching impact of poor breathing habits. Here are just a few of the health problems linked to oxygen deficiency:

Chronic fatigue syndrome
Allergies and asthma
Chronic colds
Stress
Frequent infections
Depression
Anxiety and panic attacks
Sleep problems
High cholesterol
Obesity
Arthritis and other autoimmune disorders
TMJ and other facial tension problems
Poor vision

Oxygen is needed for the functioning of every one of the seventy-five trillion cells in your body. From oxygen comes a substances that nourishes and energizes each and every cell. This substance is called adenosine triphosphate, or ATP. Dr. Hendler refers to it as the "basic currency of life." Without this spark of energy, fueled by oxygen, there is no life. The more we have, the better we feel, and the less we have, the more handicapped we are. The older we get, the more we need to draw this fuel deep inside if we are to maintain our health and well-being.

The vast majority of us were born with our naturally relaxed and instinctive deep-breathing patterns intact. Then came stress. Or, more accurately, then came the stresses of modern society and our reactions to them. The nature of stress has changed dramatically in recent history, turning our basic flight-or-fight response into a full-time job.

The flight-or-fight response is our body's way of mobilizing its defenses when under threat. As the decision is made whether to run or fight back, a number of physiological changes get us ready for action. One of them is a defensive tightening of our breathing. This strategy is great if the event is quick and physical, like, say, an attack by a saber-toothed tiger. If the incident goes on for long, this first-alert tactic rapidly begins taking a physical and emotional toll. These days, this incident is generally known as Life, and our stresses are, by and large, emotional and continual.

Tense shallow breathing becomes a habit. Millions of us breathe only into the top third of our lungs. We rarely use the bottom third, where the complete exchange of carbon dioxide for oxygen occurs. As a result, every cell in our bodies receives only a fraction of what it needs for true vitality, and nowhere more so than our eyes.

As you adjust your attitude toward breathing and develop your capacity to breathe more freely, educate yourself as much as possible. I highly recommend Dr. Hendler's book. Another with fascinating information and a beautiful presentation is Gay Hendrick's *Conscious Breathing*. He offers a wonderful selection of breathing exercises for a wide variety of problems.

I have learned over the years, however, that learning healthy breathing patterns while in what could be called a conscious, analytical, left-brained state of mind is an uphill struggle. Breathing exercises are fabulous for you, but the benefits are limited if these exercises don't also translate into deeper breathing habits on the automatic, nonthinking level. In other words, you can't remember to breathe more deeply all the time—it has to become a subconscious physical habit.

The Breathing Affirmations are for internalizing habits as

well as beliefs. As you relax and focus on your breathing, while affirming its quality, you're reprogramming your subconscious control tower to turn breathing exercises into real-life habits. You'll feel and literally see the difference.

Before you begin, close your eyes and survey how you feel. How are your eyes, your whole body, your energy level, and breathing right now?

BREATHING AFFIRMATION

Let your breathing be slow, deep, and abdominal. Use your imagination to let it feel as if your whole body is breathing.

"Breathe" your way from ten down to one.

Savor the relaxation.

Your affirmation is:

Inhaling: "Naturally deep inhalations."

Exhaling: "Complete exhalations."

Enhance the process along with the affirmation by activating even more of your creative imagination. Have a sense of the air as energy. You might imagine a tingling sensation inside as the oxygenated energy permeates every cell of your body. Or, you may visualize a color flowing in and out of you, perhaps as a light of healing white, gold, or blue. Breathe in the energy, the life force, and breathe out tension.

Do this for at least ten breaths before you count yourself up into energized alertness.

Don't you feel lighter and more expansive? More alive and energetic?

LIFESTYLE ADJUSTMENT

If you haven't already this morning, do some Stretching, yawning, and Curling. Afterward, close your eyes and focus on your face. Couldn't it be still more relaxed as well as energized? Give it a massage, at the very least on the eyebrows, the bones around the eyes, and the center of your forehead.

Good. Now your eyes can benefit even more from a breathing exercise that will get circulation into every cell of your lenses. I fervently hope you'll make it a permanent part of your everyday lifestyle, because it's a holistic workhorse. It will set your breathing pattern for the whole day and can be a fabulous energizer whenever you need a lift. It'll also loosen your hips, relax and strengthen your lower back, and tone your stomach muscles. And, just as importantly, it feels great.

I call it the Rocking Breath [illustration 7]. No doubt, it's been used forever, but it was developed for therapeutic use by the pioneer of body-centered psychology, Dr. Wilhelm Reich. Reich was ahead of his time and is still considered controversial today, but his insights reminded us to put the mind and body back where they belong—together.

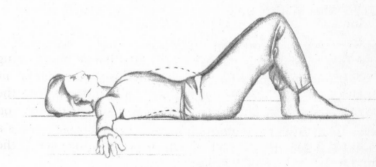

Illustration 7: Rocking Breath

Breathing is the mind-and-body link. Seeing this, Reich realized that "emotional and physical states can be altered by changing the breathing pattern." It's still a revolutionary concept for the Western mind, even though we're living proof of it on a daily basis.

Before you begin, tune inside again. The Breathing Affirmations should have you feeling pretty good, but there's more change to come. Music that you would use for swinging will help you move smoothly and rhythmically.

Lie on your back with your knees up, feet flat on the floor.

All of your breathing (as always in every exercise) will be through your nose.

While inhaling, arch your lower back off the surface beneath you while letting your abdomen balloon out. Can you slip a hand into the space under the arch of your back? If so, good. If not, know that it is especially important to keep gradually working on it.

As you exhale, pull in your stomach muscles and flatten out your lower back. That's all there is to it. Make your inhalations full and your exhalations complete. Feel, and enjoy, the smooth and gentle rocking of your hips.

Do this for twenty breaths. However, stop anytime you feel lightheaded, tightness or tingling in your fingers or face, or any other discomfort.

Keep your eyes closed and stay focused on the sensations. Then, when you are finished, stretch out and relax for a minute.

How do you feel? More energized than before? Take a look at this page without your glasses and see how your eyes responded.

Just this much breathing can revolutionize your well-being. Not that this is the end of your breathing training during this program by any means! If, however, you would like to take this exercise to greater and more stimulating heights, I again recommend Gay Hendrick's *Conscious Breathing*. Further adventures await you.

VISUAL ADJUSTMENT

First, warm up your eyes to get them ready for some intensive stretching that will open up even more circulation. Spend about two minutes swaying from side to side as in Rocking the Babies. This time, however, keep your eyes open and extend your index finger out and up as you did during yesterday's Long Swings. Keep your eyes on your fingernail and let it move right along with the rest of your body. Be aware of the background moving in the opposite direction, but don't forget to breathe and blink. When you're finished, see if you can focus on your fingernail more clearly.

The Yoga Eye Stretches [illustration 8] have helped eyesight for thousands of years. You will be stretching your extraocular muscles, the ones that control your eye movements. Working these are necessary for general visual health, and the effects reach all the way into your lenses. This is a vigorous workout, so don't overdo it if your eyes feel strain.

You'll be going through the exercise twice, once with your eyes open and then with them closed. Everything will be coordinated with your breathing, and your head will remain *still*.

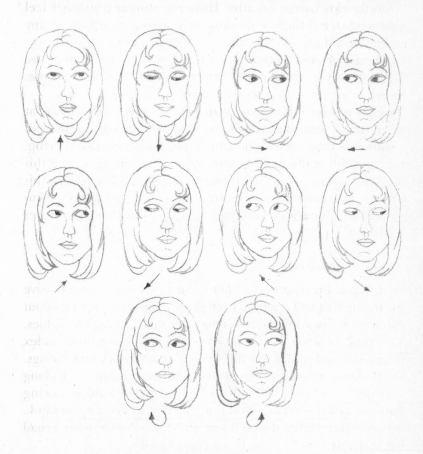

Illustration 8: Yoga Eye Stretches

Sit comfortably, back and neck straight but relaxed, eyes open.

Inhale. As you exhale, look up. Keep looking up as you take in another breath.

Exhale as you look down. Stay with that stretch as you inhale.

Exhale as you look to your left. Hold as you inhale.

Exhale as you look right. Inhale.

Stay with the breathing pattern as you make four separate diagonal stretches—up to the left, down to the right, up to the right, and down to the left.

On an exhalation, roll your eyes twice around in a circle in a clockwise direction. Inhale.

Exhale while rolling your eyes twice around in a circle in a counterclockwise direction.

Close your eyes and relax for a few moments, then repeat the entire sequence with your eyes closed.

Finally, relax your eyes with several minutes of Palming [illustration 9]. Cover your *closed* eyes with the palms of your hands, blocking out all light. Allow the darkness to soothe your eyes as you breathe abdominally.

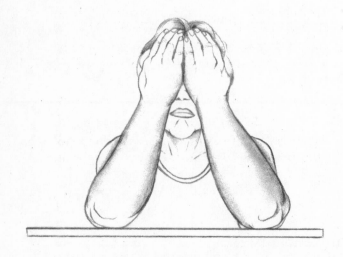

Illustration 9: Palming

Your eyes love to be palmed, especially if you first warm your hands by briskly rubbing them together. As you let the darkness envelop you, circulation opens into your eyes and your entire visual system receives an intensive and rejuvenating rest. The blacker the darkness, the deeper the relaxation. The key to achieving this is to focus on your breathing and to let go of extraneous thoughts. Whenever they come to you, just chuckle at their tenacity and bring your attention back to the pleasant feeling of your breath. You'll find that small visual and mental breaks like this will yield large rewards of clarity and well-being.

TODAY

- Be aware of how good it feels to have naturally deep inhalations and complete exhalations.
- Is there a ten-minute block of time you can set aside for some refreshing Stretching, Curling, Long Swings, and Rocking Breaths?
- Seize brief moments to stretch your eye muscles in every direction. Top them off with some Palming or a Facial Massage.
- Do the same with the Lens Flexor.
- Notice when you respond to situations by holding or constricting your breath. Take deep ones instead.

DAY FIVE

The very act of paying conscious attention to bodily functions instead of leaving them on automatic pilot will change how you age.

Deepak Chopra
Ageless Body, Timeless Mind

ATTITUDE ADJUSTMENT

Every time you consciously massage, loosen, and stretch your eye muscles, you're changing them for the better. The same goes for the cumulative effect of each conscious deepening of your breath and gentle blink of your eyes. Our attention generally starts with little bursts of awareness (Goodness, I've been holding my breath for a minute!), and eventually builds into new habits.

Sometimes, however, a shift in awareness can bring about nearly instantaneous changes. One of the most impressive turnarounds in vision and the aging process I've witnessed was primarily due to the act of conscious attention. Karla, a hyperactive journalist, was dismayed not only to be presbyopic and thirty-six, but also that her condition was progressing at a rapid rate. Indeed, the rest of her was following suit. She looked at least ten years older, and considerably more so in her shoulders and upper back, where her tension manifested in what appeared like an osteoporosis hump.

Tense breathing patterns turned out to be the core of her problem, but with an added twist: Karla smoked at least two packs of cigarettes a day. I'll be getting into smoking later, but suffice it to say that smokers generally have a much earlier onset of presbyopia than nonsmokers. The bottom line is that there is less oxygen, moisture, and nutrients going into the lenses.

I explained to Karla that I had observed her breathing patterns, and, like many smokers, it looked like the only time she took a full breath was when she inhaled cigarette smoke. Then I asked her to take a deep, abdominal breath on her own. All she could manage was a shallow gasp into her upper chest. We couldn't get past this until I finally told her to pretend she was taking a deep drag on a cigarette. Voila! Her abdomen and entire chest inflated completely.

Karla had an epiphany. Nearly everyone is surprised by the effect of breathing properly, but for Karla this was a revelation of major proportions. She had a profound insight that her smoking was a positive instinctual behavior—positive, but of course maladaptive. Still, when habitual tension patterns closed down her breathing, she had acted in the best way she knew to open it up again. I agreed with her conclusion and pointed out that the single best way to develop healthy breathing was to simply become aware of it.

Karla took my advice even more fully than I intended. No more vision lessons for her—this one would be all she'd need. She was convinced that staying aware of and opening up her breathing would take care of virtually everything. So we talked more about her breathing and tension patterns, and I gave her a few visual pointers and simple exercises, some nutritional information, and sent her off with a copy of Gay Hendrick's *Conscious Breathing*.

I never saw Karla again, but she called me three weeks later. Not even identifying herself, she burst out, "I can read tiny print, I can breathe, and I don't smoke!" I knew who it was. Indeed, Karla now knew who she was, too. "I'm a breather, not a smoker!" She had put together awareness, breathing techniques, and positive affirmations to cope with virtually every aspect of her life, from social interaction and talking on the telephone to reading and writing. Whenever she felt the urge for a cigarette, for example, she would ask herself what she wanted to get from it. The answer might be anything from relaxation to energy to confidence to love. She would then breathe deeply while affirming that she had this quality. As her self-discoveries and breathing opened, her need to smoke simply vanished.

Karla used only one vision exercise, the Finger Shift (you'll be learning this later). Before reading she would spend several minutes with it while breathing deeply and affirming, as I had suggested, "Limber lenses, clear up close." That was her entire vision program, though she had also added vitamins and herbal supplements and lots of water to her diet and joined a yoga class. I had a feeling she looked thirty-six again.

As you pay more attention to the way you use your eyes, body, and breathing when you read, you'll find counter-productive habits shifting into beneficial ones, and the print will clear.

Become consciously aware of all these things that can interfere with your vision when you read:

Holding your breath
Shallow breathing
Not blinking
Not giving your eyes frequent rest breaks
Frowning, or tightening any facial muscles
Poor lighting, either too little or glare
Slumped or imbalanced posture
Holding the page at the wrong angle—it should be parallel to
    your face, not flat on a table.

BREATHING AFFIRMATION

Let's use today's affirmation to enhance your ability to pay close
attention to how you use your eyes when you read.

After relaxing deeply with your ten countdown whole-body
breaths, and savoring the sensation for awhile, affirm for at least
ten more breaths:

Inhaling: "Conscious vision."
Exhaling: "Clear vision."

Savor the sensation again before counting yourself up,
"Awake, Alert, and Refreshed!"

LIFESTYLE ADJUSTMENT

Paying close attention to the impact of other substances you
bring into your body is our lifestyle topic for today. Before we
get to nutrition and your vision, let's open circulation into your
eyes with some warm-up exercises. Spend about five minutes
with them.

Yawn as you stretch up. Take your yawns to new heights.
Make them bigger and noisier than ever. Bring tears of circulation into your eyes!

Let your arms relax as you bring them down, but keep on
yawning. While your jaws are open all the way, open and close
your eyes four or five times. Open as wide as you can, and
squeeze tightly shut. Can you feel the extra burst of circulation
and moisture? Go through this process several more times.

Next, curl down and up four times. Each time you're hanging

all the way over from your waist, swing your head to loosen your neck—side to side, front and back, diagonally in both directions, and circles in both directions.

Now you're ready for some lifestyle information. We'll begin with a substance so vitally important that it falls into the Attitude Adjustment category, along with breathing. This is: *water!*

Let me sum up it's importance to your aging process; including that of your eyes, with another quote from Deepak Chopra:

> Not drinking enough water every day is one of the commonest conditions in old age, and although it has received almost no publicity, chronic dehydration is a major cause of preventable aging.

Like the earth, we are 70 percent water. Every cell in our bodies must be awash in water to function optimally. The brain and eyes need perhaps even more hydration than other organs. In fact, many symptoms of senility are directly linked to a lack of sufficient water. As for our eyes, their finely filtered circulation system needs extra moisture to compensate for the slowdown that comes with age. Lenses dry out easily, and they need all the help they can get.

The widely recommended six to eight glasses of water a day should be your minimum. If you take in things that dehydrate you, like alcohol, caffeine, or polluted air, you need extra water as a counterbalance. In this day and age, bottled water (though not necessarily mineral water) is generally the best choice. If you really don't like the taste of water, flavor it with a slice of lemon or lime, a dash of fruit juice, or something else you like. Your skin will glow youthfully, your elimination will be better (a great boon to your circulation!), and you'll see more clearly.

Of course, food is also crucial to our well-being, and can help or hinder our vision. Next week we'll look into the matter of specific vitamins, herbs, and other supplements for vision boosting, but first comes a look at the quality of your diet.

I want to make it clear that I am not a representative of the "food police." In fact, I think worrying about unhealthy food is probably more of a health risk than eating it; fear takes a greater toll. Still, there are some basic nutritional facts about food and its role in vision.

The general rule of thumb is that the more meat, fat, sugar, refined flour, and assorted toxins there are in your diet, the more your sight is going to suffer. Anything that weighs you down, clogs up your arteries, or depletes your natural energy is going to have a similar, but magnified, effect on your vision. The older we get, the more this holds true.

You don't have to make radical changes in your diet to see improvement in your eyesight. However, I must say that I have observed that vegetarians with a particular combination of diet and attitude almost always have great success in vision work. Their diet relies heavily on vegetables, fruits, nuts, beans, rice, and tofu, and is very light on cheese and other dairy products (they often take calcium supplements). At the same time, they have an easygoing attitude toward their lifestyle. They live this way because it feels good, not because they fear for their health. In fact, if they get a hamburger craving, they satisfy it, guilt free.

Giving up meat is not a prerequisite for vision improvement, but lots of fatty meat puts a real damper on our circulatory flow. For our vision and all-around health, the older we get, the better it is to think of heavy meats as condiments rather than main courses. Protein is essential to healthy vision, but it is best obtained from lighter meats and fish, nuts, and combinations of beans and grains. Soy products, especially tofu (there really are creative ways to prepare it!), have the added benefit of being cancer-fighting agents.

Certain foods, particularly among the fruits and vegetables, are absolute powerhouses of visual nutrition. The chemical substances in them will be outlined in the later section on vitamins, herbs, and minerals. At this point, I'll simply list a selection of some of the delicious morsels that have the special nutrients necessary for limber lenses.

avocados	all citrus fruits,
strawberries	especially grapefruit
spinach	pumpkin seeds
kale	broccoli
collard greens	asparagus
carrots	sweet potatoes
peaches	whole grains
sunflower seeds	beans
walnuts	

Citrus fruit have some special qualities to note. Grapefruit are potent medicine, but can sometimes have extremely dangerous interactions with certain drugs. If you are taking prescription drugs, check with your pharmacist to see if there will be a conflict. All citrus fruit have many of their most important nutrients, especially bioflavinoids, in the white pulp of the rind. Peeling and eating a grapefruit like you would an orange isn't exactly dainty, but it's the healthiest way to go. It's also worth a try to nibble the insides of orange and tangerine peels—you may be one of us who find this quite a tasty treat.

Dark leafy green vegetables are important for your lenses, but they are also proving to be therapeutic for other conditions of the aging eye. Spinach, kale, and collard greens have been shown to not only prevent macular degeneration, they are also capable of reversing the condition. Macular degeneration, a deterioration of the central vision that we need for reading and other images not in our periphery, is the leading cause of blindness for people over the age of fifty-five. Your best protection against it is to make these foods a regular part of your diet.

Actually, there is one more important protection from both macular degeneration and early as well as rapidly progressing presbyopia. If you smoke, you are much more threatened with these problems. Smokers have a more than 50 percent higher rate of macular degeneration than nonsmokers, as well as earlier and more advanced presbyopia. There is even a rare condition known as tobacco amblyopia, in which the protective coatings of the optic nerves are destroyed. Interestingly, the resulting blindness reverses itself when smoking stops. Young eyes and bodies, like Karla's, rebound very quickly, but every smoker is helped by each and every reduction in the amount of smoking. Compensatory measures—more water, citrus, and dark leafy greens—also help, along with extra breathing and physical exercise.

Compensatory measures are in order for all of us. How much you need, of course, depends on how long you've been wearing glasses, how strong they are, your physical condition, and how much improvement in your vision you desire. Even if your goals involve huge changes, remember that they, too, best come about in small increments and gradual adjustments.

VISUAL ADJUSTMENT

Small increments will loosen your lenses more today while also restoring more natural vibratory movement to your eyes. Before you learn something new, get your eyes ready with three minutes of Long Swings followed by a round of Yoga Eye Stretches. This morning, set your mood with music that appeals to you.

For the first minute of swinging, close your eyes. Breathe and relax as you swing from side to side, and simply be aware of the sensation of vibratory movement in your eyes.

Then, open your eyes as you continue the movement. Stretch out your right arm and keep focusing on the fingernail of your index finger. Be aware of the opposite movement in the background.

As you swing, play with the position of the finger you're watching. Keep it out in front of your eyes but move it around— it can go higher, lower, and closer to your face. Breathe and blink while you watch this extra element of motion.

After one minute, switch arms as you continue for another minute. Try yawning as you swing. Wonderful! Now, quickly go over the Yoga Eye Stretches. Look up, down, left, right, diagonally, and around in circles, first with your eyes open and then with them closed. Breathe!

Now we'll take this farther with a small movement that is a powerful visual loosener. Dot Swings [illustration 10] are taken from an old Bates exercise which has proven its effectiveness for many decades. They are also great mental relaxers, and particularly effective in soothing away headaches. Take your glasses off, of course, even if the images become blurry.

With the first illustration (dot, line, dot) directly out in front of you, point your nose at the dot on the left of the line. Then move it across the line to the dot on the right. That's all there is to it! Your head moves slightly from side to side, as though you're saying no as your eyes slide from dot to dot.

As you do this, you'll notice that the line appears to move in the opposite direction of your swing. Cultivate this illusion—it's the essence of this exercise.

Slide back and forth about twenty times, breathing and blinking.

Then move on to the next set of dots so that you're moving your head and eyes up and down across the horizontal line.

Next, repeat with each of the diagonal lines and dots.

Repeat the entire process two more times with your eyes *closed* while you continue to physically move your nose from dot to dot. Your goal is to visualize a perfectly sharp and clear image and to "see" the illusion of the line moving in the opposite direction of your swing.

The first time through, envision the dots and lines the same size as on the page. On the second repetition, imagine that they are only half that size and only about twelve inches in front of you. Yes, the movement of your head and the line is very small, but that's what we're after here.

Finally, let it go, and keep your eyes closed a few more moments while you notice the subtle but distinct effects.

Can you feel how your neck has relaxed and vibratory energy has come into your eyes? About half the people I work with experience a burst of visual clarity after their first practice with this exercise. What about you?

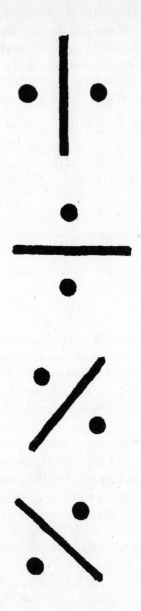

Illustration 10: Dot Swings

You can practice these for a few moments now and then throughout your day whenever you have a chance to close your eyes. If you spend a lot of time at a desk, copy the page so you can have it handy for open-eye practice as well.

TODAY

- Pay close attention to the way you use your eyes.
- Also pay attention to what you put inside your body.
- Increase your water intake.
- Accompany your yawns with alternately squeezing your eyes shut and opening them as much as possible.
- Stretch your eyes and your spine.
- Take a five-minute break from everything. Palm your eyes, feel your whole body breathing, and relax into the darkness.

DAY SIX

Whatever is flexible and flowing will tend to grow, whatever is rigid and blocked will wither and die.

Lao Tzu
Tao Te Ching

ATTITUDE ADJUSTMENT

A research study conducted nearly three decades ago is one of my favorite examples of just how flexible our visual system can be. It involved eye-and-brain communication in the transmission and interpretation of electrical impulses from the retina to the visual cortex.

The retina, which is extraordinarily complex and not fully understood, is made up of multilayered brain cell tissues. Its light-sensitive photoreceptors, the rods and cones, are chemically stimulated by the incoming light reflected off the objects we are viewing. The lens not only directs the light to the retina, but its refraction also turns the image upside down, just as a camera lens does. The moment this topsy-turvy information strikes the 127 million or so light receptors, it then rockets back through the millions of optic nerves to the rest of the visual cortex at 423 miles per hour. Here, still within a fraction of a second, the visual center puts all these nerve impulses together, turns them over, and we "see," right side up, what's out there.

This particular study focused on what would happen visually if the brain received images in a different way. Precisely, right-side up. An intrepid researcher was fitted with a special pair of prism glasses that reversed the incoming light recorded by the retina. Would he now see everything upside down, or would his brain rise to the challenge and flip them back over into a coherent interpretation of what was out there? He looked through these glasses, and reality was reversed. No instantaneous adaptation occurred.

The question now became: Would a little time and effort enable his visual system to make the necessary adjustments? Could visual flexibility be a learned skill, one we can activate when it benefits our survival and sense of well-being? You bet. It took about a week, but his willingness to change what had become an inappropriate as well as inconvenient view of his world prevailed. His brain made the adjustments, turned the images over, and the researcher's world was rightside up again.

I read of this study in an optometry textbook, and true to "pure" science, there was no mention, and most likely no note taken, of the purely subjective emotional reactions and responses of the man behind the prism glasses. However intense these may have been, his willingness to change his perception clearly carried him through the uncomfortable period of adjustment.

Returning flexibility to your lenses is certainly a far less daunting feat than overturning your whole world view, yet, at the same time, it can be just as much of a challenge. After all, there's the added physiological necessity of turning back the clock, as well as the mental task of overcoming the conditioning that says it can't be done.

I have yet to work with a client who achieved the return of

visual flexibility and maintained it without a corresponding improvement in attitudinal outlook. A "hardening of the attitudes" is contrary to the limbering of the lenses through which we look at life. Brains which send out the strongest signals for visual adaptation seem to have a similar emotional flexibility to live as a whole.

At this point, you are perhaps wondering, as I long did, about all the people who retain clear vision and yet are negative thinkers and set in their ways and opinions. The mysteries of the visual process are at work here. Still, it's safe to say that we each carry our stresses, including the aging process and its impact, in different ways. The parts of ourselves that break down as time goes by reflect the complex interaction of personality, environment, and genetics.

We can exert some control over these factors, but it's with our power of mind that we really influence our well-being. Let today's Breathing Affirmation enhance the flexibility of your attitudes as well as your eyes.

BREATHING AFFIRMATION

We'll use just two key words from today's quotation. "Flowing" will stand for the open flow of circulation you want to stimulate into your eyes, and "flexible" includes your whole body, as well as your lenses and attitudes.

First, there are your ten countdown breaths, each one there to assist you in letting go of externals and going inside. Every time you imagine your whole body breathing, feel like you're moving downward, or just experiencing relaxation, you can be sure you're entering into a state of mind receptive to the affirmation.

Enjoy the peaceful feeling, and then spend at least ten more breaths mentally repeating:

Inhaling: "Flowing."

Exhaling: "Flexible."

Savor your relaxation, the good feeling of knowing you're becoming more flowing and flexible. Then count yourself up into relaxed, alert energy. Stretch and enjoy some good yawns.

LIFESTYLE ADJUSTMENT

Today's lifestyle information will have its accompanying exercises in the Visual Adjustment section, so, as we did yesterday, let's warm up physically with some of what you've already learned.

First, loosen your spine and begin breathing using some Rocking Breaths. For fifteen full inhalations and exhalations, let your hips move fluidly as your arch and flatten your lower back.

Then give yourself a full Facial Massage. Pay special attention to any places that feel tight, and yawn often. When you're finished, don't forget to observe the effects on your vision as well as your mood.

Our quotation today reminds us that "whatever is rigid and blocked will wither and die." So, therefore, will the vast majority of life forms, including us, without one of our most abundant but often abused or neglected resources. Like water, this is a topic so important it could also be an Attitude Adjustment. It gets a quote from the highest source:

> Let there be Light.
>
> God

God didn't mean artificial light. Life and vision depend on light, and they flourish best in the presence of sunlight. Surely, you already know that sunshine contains vitamin D, crucial for our absorption of calcium, but you may not be aware of its other health benefits.

Twenty-five percent of the light that enters our eyes does not continue on to the visual cortex, but is relayed from the retina to the hypothalamus. This is the brain's "master gland," and it regulates the functioning of our nervous and endocrine systems. This control tower is literally fed by light, but not all light is equally nutritious.

For a detailed and fascinating account of the importance to our health of all the colors in the light spectrum and different ultraviolet wavelengths, I urge you to read pioneer light researcher John Ott's 1976 ground-breaking book *Health and Light*.

His research is impressive, and his personal experience of having arthritis spontaneously vanishing after he broke his glasses is inspiring.

It's almost as if, like plants, we photosynthesize in the presence of sunlight. Our health, mood, and vision all bloom in the right light, which brings me, inevitably, to the unavoidable subject of our depleted ozone later and the current antisun hysteria. For every one of us gently reminding you of the benefits of *moderate* amounts of soft sunshine, it seems that there are one hundred others shrieking that you must wear sunglasses, a hat, and slather yourself with sunscreen if your are *ever* exposed to the sun. But we are not moles, and the ozone layer is not so depleted that we need protection from all sunlight. Sunburn and frequent exposure to hot sun and glare are certainly dangerous, but we have come to the classic situation of "throwing the baby out with the bath water."

There is no shortage of researchers and reasonable doctors, including eye doctors, who share my opinion. We are in general agreement that at least twenty minutes to an hour of *gentle* morning or late afternoon sun a day is essential for good health and well-being. (If you have to tip your head back to face directly into the sun, it's high enough in the sky to be in the danger zone.)

If this were a real workshop, we would begin each day with the "sunning" exercises you will learn in the next section. In fact, we would spend as much time as possible outside, even while the sun is at its highest if the temperature's comfortable. Not in direct sun, of course, but where it's safely filtered. If we had a good solid week or more together, every one of you would feel better as well as see better, and the sun-impoverished among you would blossom the most magnificently.

If you had considered yourself photophobic—overly sensitive to light—you might be amazed at your transformation into a light lover. You'd be comfortable in bright light, and your sunglasses would become relegated to their rightful place as emergency protective measures.

Ah, sunglasses. Nearly all glass interferes with the healthy wavelengths of sunlight we need, but sunglasses are the worst offenders. The cheap ones ought to be illegal. They do not afford enough protection from the ultraviolet rays that are dangerous in excess. In addition, they actually let in more ultraviolet rays than you would get with your naked eye, because the darkness expands your pupils. Photochromic lenses (the kind that darken in the presence of light) don't get this dark, and they cause eyestrain indoors because any light keeps them from being truly clear.

When you're at the beach, out on the water, around snow, or driving when the sun reflects off oncoming windshields and chrome, you've got the kind of glare that is an emergency situation, and the right sunglasses are your best line of defense. In these cases you want high-quality, optically ground glass lenses (plastic ones often contain irregularities that bring more eyestrain), preferably in a neutral gray tint. The high cost of designer names grates on me, but Ray-Ban, Vuarnet, Serengetti, and the other trendy brands are indeed good sunglasses.

Of course, lack of sun is as much of a problem as overly intense light. What do you do if you live where the sun rarely shines or you truly cannot get out into it? Use the best artificial light you can—not the potentially dangerous lamps intended for suntanning, but full-spectrum incandescent or fluorescent lights. These are now widely available (though rarely in markets), and I highly recommend you replace as many of your old bulbs with them as possible. If you can't find any in lighting stores or catalogs, your next best bet is the type for growing plants indoors.

Natural sunlight and fresh air are no less important to our health and vision then water and food, and are even more vital to our sense of well-being. The older we get, the more this holds true. Don't fall into a sedentary, housebound trap. The darkness is a place to wither and die. Live in the light!

VISUAL ADJUSTMENT

Give your eye muscles a good warming up with a set of Yoga Eye Stretches, first with the eyes open and then with them closed. Relaxing background music, as well as the Sunning (to come), will help them. If your eyes feel tired after the stretches, palm or massage around them before going on.

Sunning was developed as a vision exercise by our esteemed Dr. Bates. Since then, we disciples have been adding more variations, and you are likely to come up with some of your own. In addition to being sure the sun is gentle and low in the sky, there are only two rules that have to be followed. One is to keep your eyes *closed*. The other is to keep your head moving. Of course, you also have to keep breathing—but you knew that already, didn't you?

If actual sunlight is not available or too high in the sky, you can use a light bulb. A 150-watt floodlight or incandescent full-spectrum bulb are the best choices. Any incandescent light will do, but fluorescent light is too soft for our purposes. However, *do not* use a heat or sunlamp.

In today's Sunning, which can be done sitting or standing, your body will remain still while your head moves. However, anytime you swing or sway outdoors you can turn it into Sunning by merely facing the sunlight and continuing with *closed* eyes. By the way, whenever you are doing eyes-open swinging outdoors, angle yourself so that you're *not* sliding your open eyes directly across the sun.

There is an unfortunate misconception among eye doctors not fully familiar with vision training that we are lunatics who tell people to stare at the sun. As you discover the benefits of proper Sunning, please share your experience with others and help clear up the confusion!

If you will be using artificial light for your Sunning, have it no higher than eye level, and sit or stand about three feet away from it. Relaxing background music will set the mood and help you maintain your concentration during this simultaneous relaxation and stimulation of your entire visual system.

Face the sun with your eyes closed, and let its soothing warmth relax your face, neck, shoulders, and whole body for a few moments. Be open to the gentle healing energy of the sunshine.

Now, begin turning your head from left to right, as if nodding no, smoothly and easily.

As your head goes back and forth, notice that even behind your closed eyelids you can detect the apparent motion of the sun moving in the opposite direction of your swing.

Time your breathing and movement together, inhaling one direction and exhaling the other, for about one minute.

Then, for the next minute, change the direction of your head motion so that you are moving it up and down across the sun.

Next are diagonal movements across the sun, first from up to the left and down to the right, and then vice versa.

And then on to making circles around the sun, both ways, of course.

Again, completely relax into the soothing sunlight. Notice how good you feel through your face, eyes, head, and neck, throughout your whole body and in your mood.

Now that everything has relaxed and loosened, we'll move on to what's known as Sun Sandwiches, which will train your iris muscles to respond more spontaneously to changes in illumination.

Turn away from the sun, and palm your eyes for three long and deep breaths. Think black, relaxing into the darkness.

For your next three breaths, take your palms down and face the sunlight again, still keeping your eyes closed.

Alternate back and forth five or more times.

Keeping your eyes closed, relax into the sunlight again. Can you let every muscle, especially those in your face and around your eyes, loosen even more?

Our final Sunning exercise in this series is called Flashing [illustration 11], which stimulates healthy retinal activity.

With your fingers spread apart, wave your hands back and forth across each other in front of your closed eyes. As your fingers move rapidly up and down past one another, you will see visual patterns from the interplay of dark and light. Let these dance and play on your eyes while you do this for about one minute.

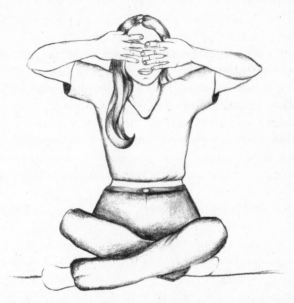

Illustration 11: Flashing

Finally, cover your closed eyes with your palms for at least two minutes, sitting or lying down with your elbows supported. As you Palm, let your whole body feel like it's breathing, and relax into the darkness. Notice how the darkness grows as time passes. You may want to enhance the darkness by imagining that pieces of black velvet are being laid, one at a time, on top of the backs of your hands. The darker the black you see, the deeper your visual relaxation.

When you are finished, keep your eyes closed so they can readjust to light behind your closed lids for about ten seconds. Blink softly when you open them.

How do you feel? How do you see up close? Does everything around you look more fresh and bright? I would say that if my clients had to vote for their single most favorite and effective exercise, Sunning would come up the winner. Even small snatches of sunshine on your closed lids when you consciously relax will bring circulation into your eyes and lenses.

TODAY

- Think of yourself as flexible and growing, like a healthy plant in the sunlight.
- Even if only brief moments are available, lift your closed eyes to the sunshine as often as possible.
- Stretch, yawn, and curl up and down.
- Drink an extra glass of water, and eat something really good for you.
- Give your eyes an extra break from reading with Dot Swings.
- When under stress, breathe!

DAY SEVEN

The best exercises for you are the ones you will do.

Edgar Cayce

ATTITUDE ADJUSTMENT

On the last day of each week it's time to review, to stop and take a look at how the week has gone, reflect on the ideas and activities, assess the progress in your vision, and spend a little time with the exercises you enjoy the most. In a real workshop, it's also the time when the group would share experiences, and I'd clear up any questions and get feedback. If you've been doing this program on your own and without much outside support, this is an especially good time to remember that even though others are not visible, you are part of a large group of people with similar goals and experiences.

So let's look at the key thoughts and attitudes you've been considering and working with this week. As you go over the quotations, consider how you felt about them at first, how much you used and thought about them during the week, and any ways in which these feelings have changed. When you come to each Breathing Affirmation, go over it with several long breaths, and see how it sits with you now.

1. "Because the mind influences every cell in the body, human aging is fluid and changeable, it can speed up, slow down, stop for a time, and even reverse itself."
   Inhaling: "Aging can slow down."
   Exhaling: "And reverse itself."

2. "You'll see it when you believe it."
   Inhaling: "I believe."
   Exhaling: "My vision is regenerating."

3. "Belief creates biology."
   Inhaling: "I am creating."
   Exhaling: "Younger vision."

4. "He lives most whoever breathes the most air."
   "Breathing is the key that unlocks the whole catalog of advanced biological function and development."
   "Breathing in, I calm my body and mind.
   Breathing out I smile.
   Dwelling in this present moment,
   I know this is the only moment."
   Inhaling: "Naturally deep inhalations."
   Exhaling: "Complete exhalations."

5. "The very act of paying attention to bodily functions instead of leaving them on automatic pilot will change how you age."
   Inhaling: "Conscious vision."
   Exhaling: "Clear vision."

6. "Whatever is flexible and flowing will tend to grow, whatever is rigid and blocked will wither and die."

Inhaling: "Flowing."
Exhaling: "Flexible."

What have been your experiences during the Breathing Affir-mations each day? Have you been able to imagine the sensation of your whole body breathing? Are you able to relax a little more with each number that you count down? During the countdown, are you able to maintain your concentration and the affirma-tions? Are you fully entering into the process, or doing it mechanically?

Be "entering the process," I mean feeling your level of relaxation increase and a sense of being in your own little world, even though you are most likely very aware of anything happen-ing around you. There are not mandatory rules, but if you're experiencing the downward sensation as you count down, or your body as if it is breathing, or just peaceful comfort, you're definitely on the right track.

Everyone's different, and I've heard a wide variety of descrip-tions of this mind-and-body state. A few examples are: inside a cocoon of peace, wrapped in a down comforter of relaxation, light and floating, pleasantly heavy and lazy, going deep inside the self, in another world, or just relaxed. How would you describe it? If the process is a struggle for you, my best advice is to relax your expectations and keep on practicing. Nothing strange is meant to happen, just a return to a natural state of peaceful well-being.

BREATHING AFFIRMATION

Practice again right now. Look at the Breathing Affirmations from this week, and choose one to repeat today. The one you feel you need the most work on would be an excellent choice. On the other hand, you could certainly go with the one you enjoy the most. Keep the Edgar Cayce quote in mind—what you are willing to do is always the best choice.

LIFESTYLE ADJUSTMENT

How have you been doing with the Lifestyle Adjustments? Let's look at the exercises first. As you look at the list, which are your

favorites? How do you feel during and after them? Now and
then, have you been able to work any or all of them into your
daily life? Are any a challenge? Have you been getting out and
enjoying the sunshine? Does your breathing seem more deep
and relaxed?

Yawning, Stretching, and Curling up and down while
   breathing deeply
Neck looseners while hanging forward and down
Abdominal breathing
Facial Massage
Rocking Breaths

This morning do a little of everything, but take less time than
you normally would with each one, and work your way down the
list. If you haven't been using any background music, this would
be a good time to experiment, especially if you're not already
thoroughly enjoying the "exercises," or having any trouble
maintaining your concentration. I'd recommend Pachelbel's
Canon in D.

Are you more limber than you were a week ago? Isn't it a delight
that just a few minutes of gentle movement can leave you feeling
relaxed and energized? Making small adjustments in your
lifestyle rather than attempting huge changes is all that it takes
to achieve your desired improvements. I hope that even those
among you who regularly do another exercise remember that
the flexibility and circulation into your eyes that this program
provides are just as important.
   During this day, see if you can find small regeneration breaks
in your daily schedule for each of the exercises. Reflect on how
you feel about each one. It's fine to have favorites; you're going
to benefit most from that which you enjoy. However, be aware of
any reasons you may have for avoiding any of them. Sometimes
obstacles are really signposts drawing your attention to where it
needs to be most.
   How's the rest of your lifestyle? Have you made any dietary

adjustments, if you needed them? These are important, but remember to go easy on yourself. Research is finally paying attention to this, and getting upset and berating ourselves for our health habits appears to be as bad as the offending substances. Negatives beget negatives, so focus on positive reinforcement. Congratulate yourself heartily for every extra glass of water, fruit, and vegetable, and forgive your little transgressions. Patience, perseverance, gradual adjustments, and a good sense of humor are your best tools for change.

Your Breathing Affirmation process is also a powerful tool you can use to make lifestyle adjustments. Create one that specifically applies to your desires—for more water, healthy food, enjoying the exercises, stopping smoking, or reducing your caloric intake.

The one rule for an effective affirmation is to use positive terms. The idea is to reinforce the desired alternative. To say to yourself, for example, "I don't want a hamburger," sends the message of "hamburger" to your subconscious brain. On the other hand, "I enjoy eating spinach" is a positive alternative. State how you want to feel or behave, even if it stretches reality a bit at first. For instance, if you're not a fan of water yet, go ahead and tell yourself that you like its taste and enjoy those eight glasses a day. It may take a while to sink in, but enough repetition will get the message through.

VISUAL ADJUSTMENT

Your eyes are younger than they were a week ago. With every exercise and visual activity you've engaged in, your lenses, ciliary muscles, and entire visual system have made some adjustment to greater fitness and flexibility.

Let's look at everything together:

Long Swings, including watching a finger move in and out
The Lens Flexor
Rocking the Babies
Yoga Eye Stretches
Palming

Dot Swings
Sunning

Which are your favorites? How often during any given day are you able to fit in a few moments of visual relaxation or stimulation? Are you experiencing bursts of clearer vision after practicing any one or a combination? It's a little early to expect clarity if you've been wearing reading lenses for a long time, but I would still expect that many of you are already seeing at least occasional improvements.

Have you found that Palming relaxes and refreshes your eyes? This deceptively simple procedure has remarkable restorative powers. The warmth and darkness gives our eyes a unique opportunity for complete relaxation. They get more needed rest and recuperation during Palming than when we are asleep. Many of us take our tension to bed with us, and our eyes as well as other parts of the body often hold on to this all night. Moreover, while the rapid eye movements that accompany dreams may be necessary for our emotional growth, they certainly aren't restful for our eyes. The more often and longer you palm the better. Try setting aside fifteen or twenty minutes now and then, and you'll get the benefits of a fabulous mental and visual vacation.

As with the Lifestyle Adjustments, today's vision session consists of working your way through the list in a brief review of each skill. Remember to breathe and blink and stay completely focused on what you're doing. Let this focus be alert but relaxed. Once again, music really helps, so try some if you haven't already. Music that you swing to is perfect. You'll concentrate better, the time will go faster, and the rhythm and your mood will increase the effectiveness of the exercises.

Before you begin, notice how well you can see print without glasses. Compare this to a week ago. Can you read without your glasses? How far away do you have to hold a book in order to see the print? If you're reading with glasses, are you able to bring the page closer than before? Could you do with a weaker prescription? Do you have one yet? Now, spend a total of five to ten minutes on all the vision exercises so far. If you feel like doing them in a different order than they're listed, go for it!

Without your glasses, look at a printed page again. How did your vision respond to an overall relaxation, stimulation, and retraining session? Do your eyes feel refreshed or tired? If they need more rest, palm for a few minutes, and top this off with some massaging of your face and eye areas.

TODAY

- Compare your vision and attitudes on aging now to one week ago.
- Let your favorite or most needed affirmation play through your mind.
- Yawn a lot!
- Drink extra water and eat something good for you.
- Try to fit in a few minutes of every physical and visual exercise.

DAY EIGHT

> Gerontophobia is ingrained in all of us, including the elderly.
>
> Ken Dychtwald
> *The Age Wave*

ATTITUDE ADJUSTMENT

Even if you're not technically part of the post World War II baby boom generation, you may still have "gerontophobia"—the fear of aging. I'm about four months too old to be an official member, but I feel that I belong to this group that created the "youth culture" which has dominated America, indeed much of the world, even before we came of age in the turbulent sixties.

Self-centered by virtue of our very numbers, nearly seventy-seven million strong in the United States alone, we redefined the parameters of age, creativity, sexuality, wisdom, power, beauty, and usefulness. The "generation gap" signified our distaste for all that was old. "Distaste" is an understatement; "revulsion" is more accurate. We didn't even trust anyone over thirty—what a joke that became on that milestone birthday!—and the mere thought of truly old people made our collective skin crawl. Aging signaled failure, decay, uselessness, and death, and we became downright phobic about it.

Interestingly, at the same time we took to the jogging trails and various health regimens to immortalize our youth, presbyopia began cropping up earlier than it had in the past. Granted, computers and other environmental factors have put an additional strain on our visual systems, but it may very well also tie in to the concept of one's self-gerontophobia.

Dr. Bates theorized that the underlying cause of most vision problems was mental tension. Today we expanded this concept to include an emotional desire to avoid unpleasant sights. In other words, if we don't want to see something, our visual system complies and shuts down accordingly. A majority of nearsighted people, for example, report responding to events before and during the time their sight first blurred with an attitude of fearful withdrawal. Usually, this is stress in early school years or the emotional upheaval of adolescence. They didn't want to see an outside environment they found frightening or unpleasant.

If nearsightedness can be seen as stemming in part from an unwillingness to look into the distance, then we must look at the possibility that farsightedness may have some link to not wanting to look up close. I always explore this area with my clients, and many do, indeed, realize that an up-close and intimate look at themselves is something from which they have been shying away.

Here are the most often cited circumstances as causes for avoidance:

Dismay and disgust at the visible signs of aging
Feelings of failure, lack of personal satisfaction

Nothing more to accomplish
Lack of self love
Lack of loving relationships
Loss of youth, beauty, abilities, or health
Fear of death

The onset of presbyopia often correlates with events that trigger the inner desire to shut out an up-close view. This may be an immediate visual reaction or it may take about a year for the system to break down. The occurrences most often recalled are:

A birthday considered a landmark of aging
The death of a friend
Divorce or other personal problems
Becoming a grandparent
An eye doctor or parent's prediction
Difficulty at work
Health problems

Does any of this ring true for you? If so, attitude adjustment is of crucial importance! This program is intended not just for regeneration and age reversal, but also for a healthy acceptance of this phase of life.

Some of the really good news is that the generation which shunned aging is now going to lead the way to reembracing it with perhaps unprecedented vigor. There's enormous power to be wielded when you're the largest age group on the earth. As Ken Dychtwald puts it in *The Age Wave*, "The boomers redefine whatever stage of life they inhabit. They have, in fact, already begun to rebuild the later years of life in their own, more youthful image."

We are already turning aging back into the glorious, vital, and respected process it's meant to be. I see this not only in the world around me, but also in every presbyope I work with whose sight improves along with the decision that the face in the mirror is not that of the enemy. Accepting rather than rejecting or resigning ourselves to aging opens the door to reinventing it.

BREATHING AFFIRMATION

Of course, we don't want to reinforce the idea of "geron-tophobia," so let's turn it around into something more positive for today's affirmation.

After counting yourself down from ten to one along with your whole-body breathing, let your next ten breaths help you focus on the phrase:

Inhaling: "Aging youthfully."
Exhaling: "Seeing more clearly."

Keep inwardly claiming these qualities even as you breathe and count yourself back into refreshed alertness.

LIFESTYLE ADJUSTMENT

Take another positive step into youthful aging with three to five minutes of warm-up exercises.

Yawn, stretch, and curl up and down.
Loosen your spine and open your breathing with Rocking Breaths.

Good. Now it's time to learn a breathing exercise that will greatly expand your breath capacity. This is called the Full Yoga Lifting Breath [illustration 12]. Each one will bring you huge regenerating doses of oxygen, along with the added side-effect of toning the muscles around your waistline. They can be practiced unobtrusively in many situations—a great way, for example, to spend the time you're stuck waiting out traffic lights.

Before beginning, close your eyes and become aware of your breathing. Don't change it, just follow it. How much expansion do you feel? How much is in the top of your chest, and how much movement is there in the lower part of your rib cage? Try keeping your eyes closed during the exercise so all your conscious attention stays on what you are doing. All your breathing will be through your nose.

Inhale abdominally to the count of four. Pull the air all the way down and let it expand your lower abdomen like a balloon.

Hold this breath.

As you're holding it, pull your stomach in and lift it up toward your ribs. Hold for a count of eight.

Exhale to the count of eight, gradually tightening your stomach muscles to squeeze out all the air.

That's all there is to it. Relax your belly and let it billow out as you breathe in.

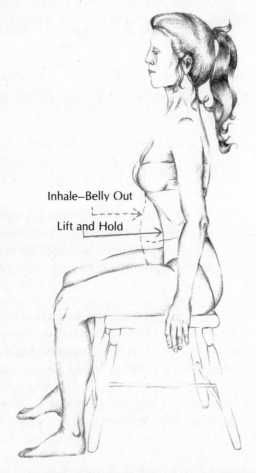

Inhale—Belly Out

Lift and Hold

Illustration 12: Full Yoga Lifting Breath

Keep on going for ten breaths. (As always, modify this according to your personal readiness.)

Then, relax and breathe normally. Experience the astounding expansion of your breath capacity!

Are you amazed at how much space you have for your breath once you expand your lungs? Can you also feel the healthy work around your midsection? When can you fit in a few of these now and then? How about while watching TV? They are great for quick bursts of energy as well as building your ability to take in and utilize more oxygen.

VISUAL ADJUSTMENT

There's a big visual workout on tap for today, so let's get your eyes ready for it with some preliminary loosening.

Start off with at least two minutes of Sunning. Also feel your neck loosening as you swing your head in all directions past the sun or the light you are using. Top this off with some Flashing before Palming for ten slow breaths.

Then enjoy Long Swings for several minutes, preferably to rhythmic music. Do the first half with your arms relaxed and hanging, and the last half with your arms outstretched while focusing on your index fingernail to stimulate even more eye movement.

Now you're ready to get out both your eye patch and big ball or minitrampoline. An alternative to using the ball or trampoline is to stand on one leg during the exercises. However, don't attempt anything that would endanger you if any of these choices are impractical due to a physical or medical condition. Even while sitting or standing you can get some added movement by bouncing gently without lifting your feet off the ground, which will increase the effectiveness of the exercises. But move somehow!

As I mentioned in the Materials List, the big rubber balls widely available make wonderful furniture as well as exercise equipment. Just sitting on them and bouncing gently while watching TV, conversing, working at a desk, or even reading is terrific. Your eyes loosen, you get a fabulous internal organ massage, your circulation opens, your balance is improved, and you relax your brain as well as your body.

It's the same with the trampoline, but it doesn't have as many uses. If you use one for your vision work (i.e., play!), keep your feet on it at all times. With your knees a little bent, you can softly bounce without leaving the mat, as well as shift your weight from one foot to the other.

If standing on one leg is your choice (which can be quite a challenge when wearing your eye patch), just lift one foot off the floor far enough to activate your sense of balance. If it's difficult, stay near a wall or chair for support when necessary.

The majority of all the exercises in this program can be practiced while stationary or in motion. But do what feels right for you, although it is my experience that people who make good use of the ball or trampoline progress much faster than those who don't. And, just as importantly, they have more fun!

So, patch your left eye and get comfortable standing on the trampoline, ready to stand on one foot, or sitting on your ball (your feet should be flat on the floor and your knees just below the level of your thighs).

Keeping your feet on the surface beneath you, bounce up and down gently (or balance on one foot), and focus on your outstretched right index finger or thumb. Notice that the background moves in the opposite direction of your finger.

One by one, shift your focus in and out from your finger to fifteen different objects in the room. Can you breathe and blink at the same time?

Then, move your patch over to your right eye and repeat the whole process.

Finally, take off the patch and do the fifteen shifts of focus with both eyes. Don't forget to breath and blink.

Ah, time to rest your well-worked lenses as they incorporate what they've done. Whether you're on the ball or a chair, prop your elbows on a table and sink into the darkness of Palming. Relax and take at least twenty slow breaths—more would be better after all you've just done.

How are your eyes? And you? Energized? Could you see your fingernail any more clearly as you worked your way through this exercise? Does everything in your view look a little brighter and sharper? Can you read more easily? Working one eye at a time is highly stimulating to the whole visual system, and actually helps the eyes work better as a team.

TODAY

- Often remind yourself that you are aging youthfully and seeing more clearly.
- Can you find a few minutes here and there for some Long Swings? Stretches and Curls?
- Wouldn't your face like a massage today?
- Bounce whenever you can.
- Practice Full Yoga Lifting Breaths.
- Play with your eye patch and shift your focus from a finger to distant objects.
- Yawn!

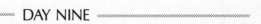 **DAY NINE**

As long as new perceptions continue to enter your brain, your body can respond in new ways. There is no secret of youth more powerful.

Deepak Chopra
Ageless Body, Timeless Mind

ATTITUDE ADJUSTMENT

We all know, of course, that hardening of the arteries can develop as we age, but did you know there's an analogous mental condition that can also crop up? It's known as "hardening of the attitudes." Optometrist Jacob Liberman's statement that "our eyesight is simply a reflection of our view of reality," means that we see the way we think. If our thinking is not flexible, our lenses most likely won't be either.

This doesn't mean that we have to abandon our convictions and ideas and adapt to every fad and fantasy that comes along. Adaptability doesn't mean letting go of what is truly valuable, but rather, as Deepak Chopra has said, it is "most simply defined as freedom from conditioned response." When we're willing to reconsider and reevaluate our beliefs and behaviors instead of making automatic, knee-jerk responses, there is an opening of energy into our physical body, including our eyes.

I have often seen the release of rigid attitudes precede a new flexibility in vision. Clara, a forty-four-year-old single mother of two teenage girls, is an excellent case in point. It so happened that a doubling of her reading prescription came about shortly after the time her sixteen-year-old daughter Leah defiantly announced that she was pregnant and intended to keep the baby.

Clara considered herself a liberated but frustrated woman, and she had spend sixteen years trying to warn her daughter not to fall into a similar fate. Clara saw her lack of a college education as a lifetime sentence to menial office work, and she wanted more for her children. Her lectures to them on the importance of good grades and going to college were the background music on which they were raised, along with admonishments to date only boys who were "going somewhere."

When Leah informed her that she was also going to marry the father of her child, a boy Clara disliked and had forbidden Leah to see, Clara really hit the roof. She ranted and cried about the boy's lack of work ethic, about ruining her life, about all she had worked for, about abortion as the only sane choice. All to no avail.

Clara didn't attend the wedding, and she had never seen her six-month-old grandson. It didn't matter to her that the trio was happy, and her son-in-law was achieving success, as his welding skills created metal sculptures that were selling at craft fairs.

This was not a career, this was indulging in artsy-craftsy, hippie stuff. Clara nursed her anger and resentment, and forbade her younger daughter to date at all.

Clara actually came to me for hypnotherapy work on the high blood pressure she had also developed during this interlude. She didn't respond to direct hypnotic suggestions to alter this until we began to more fully look at her life situation. Once she realized she was attempting the impossible task of trying to live through her daughters, everything changed.

Clara enrolled in college to become a CPA (certified public accountant). She let her daughters have their own dreams. Her blood pressure dropped. She had a few tough moments with the realization that part of her rejection of her grandson was related to the issue of aging because she was now a grandmother. I supplied her with a list of reading recommendations, and she emerged not only proud of her age but also younger in spirit. She has a wonderful relationship with her grandson now, though she is still not thrilled with being called "granny."

Clara's interest in vision improvement began after her first month of school. She'd forgotten her glasses one day, and later she was unable to read the poorly scrawled notes she'd made during her classes. It grated on her sense of independence.

Being used to a rather sedentary lifestyle, Clara found it hard to get herself to do the physical exercises I recommended. Her vision improvement efforts had only moderate results until I convinced her to join a yoga class offered at her college the hour before her normal starting time. The group atmosphere gave her the boost she needed. Her new flexibility, coupled with plenty of inversion exercises, increased the flow of circulation into her eyes, and her ability to read without glasses changed dramatically. Within a month she was entirely free of them.

If you're holding on to attitudes that restrict your mental or physical flexibility, reexamine them. If you already experiment with new ideas and experiences, keep it up. Among my oldest clients who've achieved the most impressive results, I can fondly recall a seventy-year-old man who took up in-line skating, a great-grandmother who mastered a computer program I couldn't begin to understand, and a seventy-four-year-old man with two goals for his seventy-fifth birthday—to do a headstand in yoga class and play bridge without his glasses. He accomplished both. New challenges and ideas clearly keep us vital at any age.

BREATHING AFFIRMATION

Relax deeply as you breathe your way down from ten to one. Then set your mental attitude for today with ten mental repetitions of:

Inhaling: "New perceptions."

Exhaling: "Younger vision."

Savor the sensations for a bit before counting yourself up into alert enthusiasm.

LIFESTYLE ADJUSTMENT

Get yourself going by doing some invigorating stretching, yawning, and curling. While you're hanging over, loosen your neck by gently swinging your head front and back, left and right, and around in circles.

I call today's new lifestyle exercise Breathing Rolls [illustration 13]. You'll be getting a wonderful overall stretch as you limber up your spine and shoulders and greatly deepen your breathing. This is one of my personal favorites. The graceful coordination of movement and breathing gives it a meditative quality that clears the mind while energizing the body. I must give credit to Gay Hendrick's *Conscious Breathing* for the arm rolling part of this exercise, which expands on the traditional yoga approach.

Lie on your back on a comfortable surface. Take a few moments to close your eyes and make a mental survey of how you feel at this point. How expansive is your breathing? How does your back feel?

Stretch your arms out in a T position.

Bring your knees toward your chest, and then lower them down to the floor near your right arm.

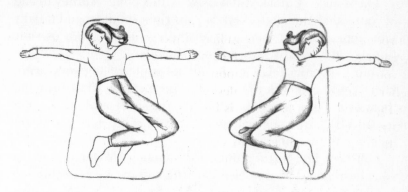

Illustration 13: Breathing Rolls

Roll your right arm over and down toward your knees. You are simply turning it so that the underside of your arm rolls forward to the floor. Notice how much mobility you have as you do this for the first time. Your shoulder joints will loosen up delightfully as you practice this exercise.

Roll your left arm in the opposite direction so that the underside comes up toward the ceiling. Again, observe how much movement there is, as well as how this feels in your shoulder and arm.

Roll your head to the left.

You are now in the full starting position. The object is to roll everything—head, arms, and knees—simultaneously and smoothly in the opposite direction. You'll keep rolling back and forth from side to side, timing everything with your breathing. Your lenses will get a little workout too.

As you inhale, move everything to the halfway position, so that at the top of your breath you're looking up at the ceiling, your knees are centered over your chest, and your arms have rolled halfway over.

As you exhale keep going, bringing your knees down on the left as your head rolls right. Your left arm is now rolled so that underside is down toward your knees and your right arm is rolled up with the underside toward the ceiling.

There's a very quick vision move at this point. At the tail end of your exhalation, look down at your right shoulder and rapidly slide your gaze out your arm all the way to the ends of your fingers, and then back up to your shoulder.

Your eyes then relax as you inhale while rolling your arms, knees, and head back to the center, then exhale while bringing them over in the other direction. There, slide your line of vision out and back up your arm as fast as you can before you begin inhaling and moving again.

Roll back and forth, aiming for as much rhythmic grace in your movements as possible. Stay with this exercise for three to five minutes, provided there's no discomfort. (Stay with it as long as you like—fifteen minutes, especially with the right music, is a sublime experience!)

Finally, stretch out again and compare how you feel now to before you began.

Doesn't this bring you a wonderful sensation of relaxed energy? If I had to pick just one exercise as my morning wake-up and intermittent refresher, this would be it. The majority of my yoga students and vision clients feel the same way.

VISUAL ADJUSTMENT

The new activity for today is an excellent one to precede vision exercises, especially those that involve the visual skill of accommodation, the shifting of focus from near to far. So we'll begin with the Hot and Cold Treatment, which will bring massive doses of nutrient-filled circulation into your lenses.

You will need two bowls of water and two washcloths. One bowl of water needs to be as hot as possible without burning your eyes. Fill the other with ice water. Cold water from the tap isn't powerful enough for this job, so add plenty of ice cubes.

The procedure is to alternate holding the hot and cold washcloths against your *closed* eyes. Propping your elbows on a table as if your were going to palm is the best position to use.

Begin with the hot water. After thoroughly wetting your washcloth, wring out the excess water and press the cloth gently to your eyelids.

Relax your face and eyes into the warmth and darkness for three minutes. As often as necessary, rewet your washcloth to keep it good and hot.

Put your mind and breath to work at the same time. With each inhalation think, "open circulation," with each exhalation, think, "flexible lenses."

At the end of the three minutes, switch over the ice-water washcloth and repeat the process.

Then continue to alternate back and forth between the hot and cold compresses, but at shorter intervals of only thirty seconds for each. Do this for another three minutes.

Do your eyes feel more refreshed and lively? Look in the mirror and you'll see the sparkle of rejuvenation. Look at the printed page without your glasses. Any immediate results? Don't force yourself to do this treatment if, for some reason, you find it unpleasant, but if it was enjoyable you can make your future sessions even longer. If you take five or six minutes for each step of the procedure, you'll gain even more benefit.

Now let's capitalize on what you've accomplished. it's time to put on your eye patch and get back on the ball (or trampoline or one leg).

Again, shift from your extended fingernail to distant objects while bouncing, like you did yesterday. If you can see your nail clearly at arm's length, bring it in toward you until it begins to blur. It won't be long until you see it clearly!

Take at least three minutes for this. Spend one minute with each eye patched, and then another using both eyes.

Finally, allow your lenses to relax and incorporate all they've done by Palming for at least ten slow breaths.

TODAY

- Remind yourself: "New perceptions" bring "younger vision."

- Relax and recharge with rock 'n roll—five to ten minutes of Rocking Breaths followed by Rolling Breaths will do it!
- Keep up the lens loosening with a minute here and there of the Lens Flexor.
- Are you drinking enough water?
- Even if you're sitting still, see how many opportunities you can find to shift your focus from your fingernail to distant objects.

DAY TEN

> A powerful agent is the right word. Whenever we come upon one of those intensely right words the resulting effect is physical as well as spiritual, and electrically prompt.
>
> Mark Twain

ATTITUDE ADJUSTMENT

A powerful agent, also, is the wrong word. I'm sure this isn't news to you, but you may not be fully aware of the subtle but profound sabotage done by hidden negatives. Even when we have good intentions, we often undermine our best efforts toward positive outcomes.

Let's say, for example, you catch yourself holding your breath when reading or in a stressful situation. What's your internal dialogue at that moment? Here are some possibilities:

"Don't hold your breath!"

"Damn, I keep holding my breath!"

"I'm never going to remember to breathe right."

The negativity in the second and third possibilities is pretty obvious. They're perfectly clear setups for a self-fulfilling prophesy, virtual commands for repeated failure even though they might have been intended to change behavior.

However, "Stop holding your breath" may seem like a positive command to break the old habit. It's not, and it's just as powerful a reinforcement of breath holding as the other two statements.

The subconscious, the seat of our habits, has to have positive commands and reinforcement to produce positive and permanent results. It needs to have a desired behavior or feeling expressed directly for two highly important reasons: it works only with the words given to it, and it tends to ignore negative ones. Therefore, when you tell yourself, "Don't hold your breath," your subconscious mind hears "Hold your breath!"

The same formula spells doom for so many of our attempts to do the right thing. Consider, for example, these common well-meant but misguided statements.:

I don't want a cigarette!
Don't strike out!
Don't play like that or you'll break your neck!
Quit dwelling on your problems!
I have to stop eating chocolate!

Take out the negatives, and you've got the message that's really being transmitted to your inner mind. Instead, it must be given the specific alternative or it will act on the information given. Positive choices to replace the ones listed above might be:

I want a deep breath!
Hit a home run!
Pay attention and play safely!
Focus on something positive!
A peach would be really good right now!

Negative ideas and concepts naturally carry as much power as individual words. Sometimes, though, we don't see them for what they can really do, and the price we pay is higher than we realize. An important case in point are jokes about aging. They bombard us from all sides, from media stereotypes to greeting cards and T-shirts to "playful" jibes at ourselves. We laugh, sometimes genuinely, but each one takes its psychological toll.

Since a sense of humor about the aging process is often essential, I've developed a strategy to enjoy the jokes and still preserve and bolster my psyche. It's a mental exercise that you may also find entertaining and useful (such things are great for keeping our brains at peak performance!).

Take, for instance, the plethora of age-insulting birthday cards and T-shirts. I happen to be guilty of finding many of these quite funny. So I go ahead and enjoy my initial guffaw, but then I get positive and creative as I continue to amuse myself by rewriting the punch line.

For example, no matter how often I see it, I am still unaccountably amused by the T-shirt that reads:

Over the hill?
What hill?
I don't remember any hill.

I laugh, and then remind myself that the last line should really read: "I've just hit my stride, and I'm cruisin' in overdrive!"

And for the greeting card that reads:

"It's your birthday." (outside)
"You can run, but you can't hide." (inside)

I just turn the inside sentiment into: "You bet I can run, and I ain't got nothin' to hide!"

If that's just too big a stretch of reality, you can always seek strength in the old adage I first heard from an eighty-year-old client: "Youth and enthusiasm will never be a match for old age and treachery."

Ah, an empowering thought indeed! And good for a chuckle, even though "treachery" would hardly qualify as an "intensely right word" for truly building self-esteem and a positive outlook on aging. For that, we could amend it to "wisdom."

Probably the single most important area to amend language is in the way we use it about ourselves. Everytime we berate ourselves, even in jest, we're adding strength to a negative self-concept. Most of us do a lot of this regarding what we perceive as signs of age. Have you, for example, ever joked about getting senile or having "early Alzheimer's" when something slips your mind? Ouch!

Verbal self-sabotage, no matter how unwitting, can have dire consequences. If you suspect yourself of falling into this trap, explore it more fully by picking up a copy of Barbara Levine's *Your Body Believes Every Word You Say*. Make this an absolute must if you have any chronic or serious health problems.

BREATHING AFFIRMATION

For now, though, consider the phrases that I have been supplying for the Breathing Affirmations. Have any contained "intensely right words" for you? Can you think of ways to rephrase any that seem to miss the mark? The more something rings true for you, the more impact it will have.

The choice of words for today's affirmation is up to you. You may want to make one up, on any topic that you feel is important. Or, you can use or amend an earlier one that carries significance for you. I suggest taking a glance at the nine we've used so far, closing your eyes, and waiting for your instincts to guide you to the right choice

Whatever your choice, don't forget to count and breathe your way into the most relaxed state you can achieve before sending the message to your subconscious.

LIFESTYLE ADJUSTMENT

Since you chose your own Breathing Affirmation today, why not your own physical warm-ups? Spend a minute with your eyes closed, surveying your body and considering what you could do to feel even better. Remember all your choices: yawning, stretching, curling up and down, massaging your face, Rocking Breaths, Full Yoga Lifting Breaths, and Rolling Breaths. Treat yourself to at least five minutes of age reversal.

Your neck is the focus of our Lifestyle Adjustment for today. The more tightness that is in your neck, the less circulation there is going into your eyes. A set of simple Neck Stretches [illustration 14] will do the trick. Stretching, relaxing, and limbering up these muscles will, of course, also give you more mobility and comfort in both your neck and shoulders.

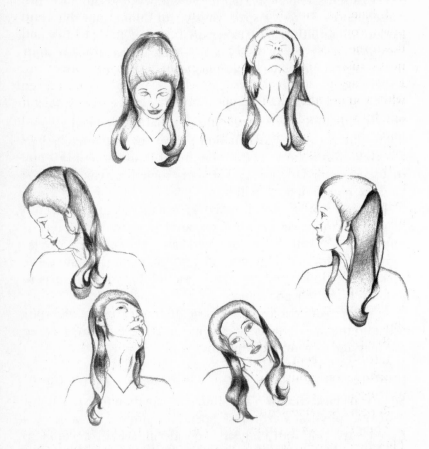

Illustration 14: Neck Stretches

These movements will leave your neck feeling wonderful and your vision clearer, provided you pay attention to one important caution. The key word for these stretches is *gentle*. Here, more of a stretch is not a better stretch. If you overstretch you stand a good chance of ending up with a headache, so take it easy and keep concentrating on your neck muscles. Your aim is to make smooth, slow movements and to relax into the stretch during the holding period.

Close your eyes as you sit upright with your head erect. Be aware of how you feel in your shoulders, neck, head, and eyes.

Inhale. As you exhale, allow your head to relax forward and down, your chin toward your chest. Feeling the stretch up and down the back of your neck, inhale again. Let it feel like your neck muscles are stretching and expanding as you breath in. Exhale again, and feel these muscles relaxing and letting go while you breathe out. Take one more breath in, and as you let it out, lift your head back to the upright position. Pause there and notice how the sensation in the back of your neck differs from before the stretch.

Turn your head and face to the left, feeling the stretching in the right side of your neck. Notice that as you inhale the stretch expands, and that as you exhale there is a release and relaxation in these muscles.

Continue on, breathing fully with each step, in the same way:

Lean your left ear over your left shoulder.

From there turn and look down at your shoulder

Then turn your face so you are looking up at the ceiling.

Turn your head so you can look back down at your left shoulder.

Bring your left ear back over your left shoulder.

Lift back to center.

Take special notice of the different sensations on each side of your neck.

Repeat the same sequence on the other side.

Then make some circles with your head, rolling to the right. They don't have to be big stretches. You can pretend you have a long paint brush on the top of your head and are painting small circles on the ceiling with it. Breathe!

Take the circles in the other direction.

Relax and compare your neck, shoulders, head, and eyes to how they felt before you began.

If your neck is stiff and creaky, you need these stretches all the more. It'll take much less practice than you might expect to soon feel, and see, a difference. Even when you don't have enough time to do the whole sequence of stretches along with focused breathing, do a little something every now and the. But gently!

VISUAL ADJUSTMENT

Now that you've stretched your neck in all directions, begin the vision session by doing the same thing with your eyes. Some lively background music with a good but easy beat would be a good accompaniment.

Breathe deeply while doing the Yoga Eye Stretches, first with your eyes open and then with them closed.

Palm for five breaths, and then massage the bones around your eyes.

Relax and loosen your eyes some more with about one minute of swaying from side to side, while either sitting or standing, and doing some Rocking the Babies with your eyes closed.

Now spend ten breaths on the Lense Flexor.

Good!

Now, back on the ball, trampoline, or one leg, and on with your eye patch. This fabulous little exercise, Color Counting, will add richness to your visual awareness in general, and stimulate the visual memory and coordination that will bring you clearer vision at every distance. Do everything with one eye at a time, and then with both together.

First, while bouncing gently or balancing, turn your head from left to right and scan the view around you. Don't make any effort to pinpoint details, just slide your eyes over everything.

Now, as you're sliding, simply be aware of the color red. As you do this, you'll notice that without any conscious effort on your part, your eyes are drawn to anything red. It will seem to jump right out at you. Observe this and keep your eyes and head moving together for four or five swings across the room. How many red objects are there? What are they?

Then move on to another color. Be aware of blue for four or five swings. Then green. Then white. Then black. Try some other colors.

Once you have gone over the distant view this way, move on to a closer one. Use a colorful photograph or magazine picture. Hold it in your hands or place it on a table or chair, close enough so the details are a little blurry. Then just slide your eyes back and forth over the page, aware of one color at a time.

Isn't it amazing how the details clear up and jump out at you when you coordinate your mind and vision? How does the printed page look now? Using the eye patch while bouncing or balancing adds an extra therapeutic boost, but you can count colors anytime and anywhere. Do it a lot!

TODAY

- Let your affirmation play through your head all day.
- Count colors!
- Stretch your neck.
- Let Dot Swings soothe your mind and loosen your eyes.
- Get out in the sunshine!
- How much water are you drinking?
- Loosen your spine and eyes with Long Swings.

DAY ELEVEN

Every good thought you think is contributing its share
to the ultimate result of your life.

Grenville Kleiser

ATTITUDE ADJUSTMENT

Whereas negatives tear us down, positives build us up. This holds true at ever level of our existence, from the emotional to the physical. I can say absolutely that the most successful vision adventurers I work with (that's how I think of us, each one of you included) are the most positive thinkers. Not just about their visual potential, but about themselves and about life.

Negativity in all its forms, from cynicism, anger, and fear, to distrust, self-doubt, and worry, puts a drain not only on the quality but even the quantity of life. We can all see this when we take a good look at the oldest people around us, but it's nice to know that research, which so often doubts the obvious until there is "data," verifies this as well. Indeed, individuals with negative outlooks, including expectations of their own life span, die at a young age three times more often than those who anticipate a long and happy life.

Good thoughts and positive expectations activate optimal physical functioning by stimulating circulation, digestion, assimilation, the immune system, and other bodily functions. Our life force flows, quite literally, when we are emotionally open and shuts down when we are constricted and defensive. Physical healing and regeneration, including visual, takes additional energy, and negative thinking is physically as well as emotionally counterproductive.

"The mind, like any other powerful force of nature, can either help or harm. It can keep us from believing that our vision can improve, or it can supply us with everything we need to improve it." This is a statement by Meir Schneider, a vision improvement teacher whose personal healing odyssey required an incredible degree of courage, dedication, and endless optimism. It took more than ten years of good thoughts and unshakable conviction for him to complete his journey from almost total blindness to fully functional vision. If you're in need of further inspiration, read his book *Self-Healing: My Life and Vision*. His story and vision exercises are also included in his marvelous contribution to the entire health field, *The Handbook of Self-Healing*.

Some happy souls seem blessed with a natural tendency to look on the bright side and expect the best. For many of us, however, this takes a concerted effort. Making the shift from negativity to optimism can often be an exercise in frustration, no matter how hard we seem to be trying. I must admit that I know this not only from the perspective of a therapist, but also from direct personal experience.

My mother, bless her heart, worried about everything. I picked up the habit, even to the point of full-blown "awfulizing," always envisioning the worst possible outcome in any given situation. It was almost a superstition, as if expecting something good would jinx its chances of occurring. As I matured I finally saw the folly in this, and embarked on the task of altering my thinking patterns. What an uphill battle! It took an accumulation of therapy, bodywork, self-help exercises, and soul-searching to provide me with tools for change.

Of course, I still backslide on a regular basis, but the practice of self-hypnosis and a few other things I've learned in recent years has kept me on the right track, as well as enabled me to better help my clients on their road to recovery. If the word "recovery" smacks of the treatment of addictions, good, because that's exactly how I mean it.

Negative thinking is addictive, not only at the habitual level but also on a chemical one. When we're involved in worry, anger, resentment, or fear, our fight-or-flight response kicks in. It may not be fun, but we get an adrenaline high. We literally become addicted to the intensity of the feeling. If we don't know how to elicit good feelings, we keep repeating what we know will at least make us feel something.

Recognizing this is the first big step, but it's still only a beginning. I cannot express it any better than this statement by John-Roger and Peter McWilliams in their wonderful book *You Can't Afford the Luxury of a Negative Thought: A Book for People With Any Life-Threatening Illness—Including Life*: "Negative thinking must be treated like any other addiction, with commitment to life, patience, discipline, a will to get better, forgiveness, and the knowledge that recovery is not just possible but, following certain guidelines, inevitable."

It's one thing to catch ourselves using negative terms, as we discussed previously, but uprooting a whole style of thinking can be a formidable task. The payoff, however, is an attitude that will foster a life of joy and satisfaction as opposed to one of struggle and disappointment. We'll get more into the specifics of how to do this as the program progresses. Meanwhile, let's lay the groundwork in your subconscious with a Breathing Affirmation.

BREATHING AFFIRMATION

Yesterday's exercise in choosing your own affirmation is something you can, of course, apply every day. If words that carry more weight for you come to mind, always substitute them for those I supply.

Go within, involve yourself fully in the relaxation and countdown procedure, and then focus on the following phrase for at least ten more breaths:

Inhaling: "Good Thoughts."
Exhaling: "Good Vision."

Own this feeling before you count yourself up into full waking alertness.

LIFESTYLE ADJUSTMENT

Let your mood and expectations be positive as you warm up your body and ocular area. Start with a Facial Massage, and then top it off with some Rolling Breaths and Full Yoga Lifting Breaths.

One of the best ways to enhance your mood and vision is to take an enjoyable walk. All walking is good for us, but a Vision Walk is special. It's a quiet stroll while you immerse yourself in a meditative visual exploration of all the details surrounding you. Your entire concentration will be on the act of observing. To completely focus on what you are doing is the essence of meditation.

When we do this, when we are meditative, we come into an emotional and physical balance that replenishes our vitality and calms our mind. This feeling of well-being enables us to respond to life in more positive ways. When you put this together with an actual vision exercise, there is an even greater boost to eyesight.

Do you have the time and a place in your life for at least a short walk? A beautiful park or the countryside would be ideal. Even an attractive residential street would be good. Where can you take your eyes to give them the closest semblance to the natural environment they were born to see? Maybe it's your own backyard.

If there aren't any natural surroundings nearby, choose the most beautiful and interesting interior that is available, a museum, perhaps, or even your favorite room at home, especially today if there's no other alternative. A video of nature scenes can even be used. Even when you are exploring details in the distance, your eyes will be making an important step toward regaining their natural confidence in their ability to successfully explore up close as well.

Brisk walks are also wonderful, but a Vision Walk is more of a mosey. It's a stroll during which you will stop often and examine your surroundings more closely. Pay attention to your breathing, blink often, and let the sun be behind you whenever possible.

First, take in the "big picture." What does the sky look like? Be aware of the perimeter of the area, and work your way in. What are the predominant colors? What are the largest forms? Let your eyes slide around their outlines. What defines this area?

Now focus your attention only on colors. Let your eyes sweep back and forth across the scene without pausing, and engage in some Color Counting. If it doesn't make you self-conscious in public; move your head along with your eyes. Think "blue" as you keep moving and scanning, and you'll notice that anything that is blue will seem to jump out at you as you slide your gaze over it. Do this a few times, and then work your way through more colors, one by one. Scan for green. For red. For yellow, Black. White. Green, in all its shades. All the colors you can think of. Each time you connect the colors visually and mentally, you are stimulating the power of both your eyes and mind.

Take this stimulation further. Go back over the colors and mentally state the identity of each object. For example, blue sky, blue dress, blue pansy, and so forth. Then, white cloud, white car, white rose, etc.

As you walk, take the opportunity to let your eyes actively seek out all the details in the scene around you. Let your eyes move with energy at different distances. Look at things nearby, look all the way down the sidewalk or path, check out what is on each side of you, look up in the sky. Examine and identify. Notice different types of plants and flowers. Once in a while, come up very close to these or other things of interest and use your near-point vision as much as possible.

If you take your Vision Walks in a familiar place, don't be surprised if you see things you never noticed before. We let our vision get lazy, and now it's time to reverse that atrophy.

Part of the idea here is to sharpen your powers of observation in every situation. You can count colors and scan for details when you're riding in a car or train, when you're gazing out your window, when you're in a store. Don't forget, however, that this is under the section, Lifestyle Adjustment. Taking a leisurely stroll with no goals other than to make it a visual meditation and to appreciate what you see will imbue the walk with an antiaging agent as well.

VISUAL ADJUSTMENT

Now it's time to give your eyes some intensive training separately, and then together, while you continue to develop your ability to focus clearly more and more close in. String Fusion [illustration 15] is a time-tested exercise employed by natural vision improvement teachers as well as eye doctors who do vision training.

You'll need your vision string set up so that it's tied to something at eye level or a little lower. A doorknob or the back of a chair will do nicely. You should have a knot tied in the string every two inches. As you read in the Materials List, I like to use brightly colored string with double knots that are easy to see. If you have trouble making out those closest to your face, you may want to color them red (or any bright color) using nail polish or a marking pen so they stand out more.

As you hold one end of the string up to the end of your nose, the entire length, between you and the other end, should be fairly still and taut. You can sit or stand for this, on your ball or trampoline. This can be done without these props, of course, but they will greatly add to it's effectiveness. Just bounce gently while you work your way through the exercise.

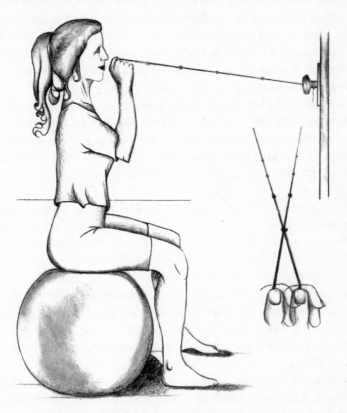

Illustration 15: String Fusion

First let's work with one eye at a time, so choose one to patch first.

Hold your end of the string up to your nose. Look out at the knot farthest away from you, and then gradually slide your gaze in towards you, knot by knot, all the way to the one closest to your face. Then shift your patch over to the other eye and repeat.

Good. Now take the patch off and use both eyes.

Look down the string to its middle. If both of your eyes are working together you'll see an optical illusion of two strings crossing at the knot you're focused on, like a big X. The reason for this is that both eyes see a slightly different image.

Demonstrate this for yourself. Close your left eye. Notice that the image of the string you see with your right eye is a bit to the left of center. Now open your left eye and close your right one. Notice that this eye sees the string more on the right side. Alternately open and close each eye, and watch the string jump back and forth.

Look at the center knot with both eyes again, seeing the two images cross in the middle, and then slide your gaze along the string to the knot farthest away from you. You will see the image of the two strings crossing wherever your eyes are focused. By the time you are out to the far end, you'll be seeing an inverted V shape.

Now, gradually slide your eyes back along the string toward your nose. The idea is to clearly see the string and knots where the string crosses all the way in to the knot closest to your nose. You'll see a V at this point. Breathe and blink as you slide in. Keep your shoulders relaxed.

Notice if and when you have trouble keeping the image of the strings crossing or seeing the string and knots clearly. This is your starting point. You'll watch your focusing ability moving closer and closer in as you progress through the rest of the program.

Whether or not you can see everything clearly, go back up and down the string five more times, up to ten if you don't feel any eyestrain. Exhale whenever you're working in a range that is a challenge.

Your eyes need a good rest after this workout. Palm and let the relaxing darkness envelope your vision for at least ten or fifteen long slow abdominal breaths. Afterward, let your hands be drawn to any area around your eyes, face, neck, or shoulders that may still feel tense and do a little massaging.

You may want to make more than one Fusion String. This way

you can leave them in places where you'll have opportunities to use them, even in brief spurts. My clients have them tied to bathroom doorknobs, TVs, refrigerators, and bedposts. If you work on a computer, tie a string nearby so you can give your eyes regular breaks from their frozen focus on the screen. This is very important work for your eyes, so do it often, but always remember to give your eyes a rest afterward.

TODAY

- Seize every opportunity for a good thought.
- Let every walk be at least in part a Vision Walk.
- Decide where to leave your Fusion String for handy workouts.
- Do a little Sunning.
- Increase circulation with a Hot and Cold Treatment.
- Stretch your neck and eyes now and then.
- Yawn! Stretching your whole body!

DAY TWELVE

How efficiently you use your "stress energy" determines your vitality and your rate of aging. The more efficiently you use this energy the greater your vitality and the slower your rate of aging—and the better you feel.

Richard Earle, Ph.D., and David Imrie, M.D.
Your Vitality Quotient

ATTITUDE ADJUSTMENT

No matter how much we engage in positive thinking, stress is always going to be a fact of life. What we can control is the way we identify and respond to it, but of course, this is often easier said than done. Outright negativity is not the only sign that we're squandering our vitality.

Let's take a look at some thought and behavior patterns that indicate a drain on our finite life force. The following list comes from Dr. Paul Pearsall's *The Pleasure Prescription*. Interestingly, he calls these "self-focusing—or selfing—factors," which gives us a good clue as to how to start changing them. Do any of these patterns that deplete "stress energy" apply to you?

1. Endless days—always feeling like there's more you should be doing
2. Distraction and forgetfulness—inability to remained focused on what's really important because there seems to be so much else drawing your attention
3. Busy going nowhere—no guiding goals or sense of purpose
4. No idea how you're doing—no feeling of support from others and no inner sense of real accomplishment
5. High responsibility with little power—believing you must take care of everything but you're not in charge of the situation
6. Everything is a big effort—even simple things
7. Never enough time—life is a race to get everything done
8. The weight of the world is on your shoulders—feeling you have to take care of everyone as well as yourself

When attitudes and behaviors like these sap our strength and resiliency, the aging process takes a greater and greater toll. It's also been my experience that the more someone exhibits these traits, the earlier they develop presbyopia.

A case in point is Dean, a forty-four-year-old restaurant owner with an ulcer, a painful sensitivity to sunlight, and very strong reading glasses. The neverending work of the restaurant business is tough, even for those who love it. Dean's attitude was ambivalent. He had grown up around this Italian family enterprise and had a real knack for it, but was oppressed by his father's ultimate control of every decision and detail. Dean felt overworked, underappreciated, angry, and frustrated.

Breathing and Sunning were the main focus of our first few lessons, and Dean found that with a few reassuring words of guidance he could relax into the sunshine instead of tensing up against it. He came to the conclusion that he had been "living like an asthmatic mole." He began to take breaks at work, something he'd never done before, to get outside to a nearby park for ten minutes of fresh air, soothing sunshine, and Long Swings or a Vision Walk. Work became more tolerable, his ulcer bothered him less, and he was able to reduce his reading prescription by one-half of a diopter.

One day I had him bring in a menu from the restaurant to use for a reading lesson, since familiar material is easier to see clearly. To my surprise, however, the menu was more difficult for him to read than what I had on hand in the same print sizes. Since he knew the menu by heart, I decided to have him close his eyes and visualize the words clearly. He couldn't do it. Even the mental image was blurry, although he'd had no problems with other visualizations. Dean laughed when I mentioned this and said, "It's probably because I hate the damn thing." Bingo!

The term *blind with rage* is no accidental metaphor. Anger literally blurs our vision, whether it's brief and intense or smoldering and ongoing. It's an energy drain and a constriction, physically as well as emotionally. Dean was angry about the menu, so he didn't want to see it.

I asked him to visualize what he'd like to see on it instead. He laughed again, but with glee instead of sarcasm, and immediately described a new color and design as well as a compendium of creative "Italian California cuisine" dishes that lightened up and expanded on the traditional offerings. As he completed the picture, I could see the beam in his eyes even through his closed lids. Then his expression melted into sadness and he began to cry.

As he spoke of his father's rebuff of his ideas, it became clear that Dean's presentation was part of the problem. He was both defensive, always assuming rejection would be forthcoming, and confrontational, insulting his father's choices as old-fashioned and fattening. I suggested a compromise, a menu with both styles of food equally offered and praised for their complimentary virtues. Since this approach had more potential than a stubborn stalemate, Dean gave it a try. With an attitude of partnership rather than competition, a beautifully done mock-up of the new menu, and a few bottles of wine as a peace offering, he succeeded in his goal and their relationship took on a new depth.

The next day, after Sunning, Dean was able to hold the menu at arm's length and read even the small print without glasses. It was several months before his vision stabilized and maintained its improvement, which happened to coincide with the "Grand Reopening" of the restaurant. It was a time of great demands and stress, but this had positive rather than negative impact once his energy was channeled positively. This works for all of us.

BREATHING AFFIRMATION

If you catch yourself making inefficient and counterproductive use of your stress energy, let today's affirmation put you back on the track of a more positive approach. Make any changes you like in the wording.

Relax more deeply with each of your whole-body breaths as you count from ten down to one.

For the next ten breaths, focus on:

Inhaling: "Clear purpose."

Exhaling: "Clear vision."

Let each breath during your count up from three to one increase your vital energy.

LIFESTYLE ADJUSTMENT

Get ready for some overall stretching by loosening up your spine with several minutes of Rocking and then Rolling Breaths.

The Leg Lift Series [illustration 16 a, b, c, and d] is a continuous series of simple yoga stretches that are wonderful for maintaining the flexible spine that is so necessary to the flow of circulation into your lenses. The whole process doesn't take more than five minutes, and you'll feel a significant improvement in your mobility and comfort. If you have any back problems, modify these moves as you feel appropriate. However, in most cases, this set of moves is a true boon to bad backs.

Find a comfortable place to lie down, supported by a thick carpet or a mat of some sort. If it meets your needs and situation, you can even do these while in bed. Close your eyes for a few moments and make a mental survey of how your body feels. Notice all the places that could be more comfortable. Notice the natural depth of your breathing. Let your eyes stay closed during the stretches, as this will keep them relaxed while, at the same time, you will have a better chance of remaining focused on the physical sensations of each of the moves.

You'll be breathing in time with your movements, so let them both be smooth and slow.

Inhale as you raise your right leg as high up as it will go. Keep it as straight as possible but also comfortable.

Hold this breath while you clasp your hands behind your leg, as high up as possible without lifting your head off the floor.

Exhale as you lift your torso up in the direction of your leg. Make it a nice stretch, not a strain. Notice how far your face is from your knee as you hold for a few moments.

Inhale as you release your leg, leaving it in the air, and lower your back down while stretching your arms out in a T position.

Exhale, and roll your head to the right, as you cross your right leg over and down to your left hand (or as close to it as you can bring it). Hold on the exhalation for as long as you can be comfortable.

Then, inhale while extending the leg back up toward the ceiling.

Exhale as you clasp your hands behind and just below your knee, and lower it down over them.

Inhale as you pull your knee in a little toward your chest, and then curl up toward it. Keep your chin down toward your chest. *Don't* strain to bring your head to your knee—this will only give you a headache. The idea is to feel and relax into the stretch brought to your lower back.

Illustration 16a, b, c, and d Leg Lift Series

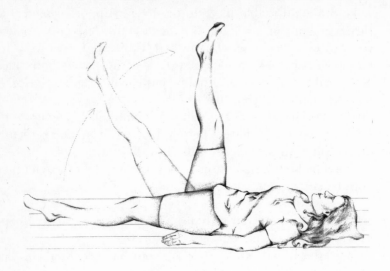

Illustration 16a

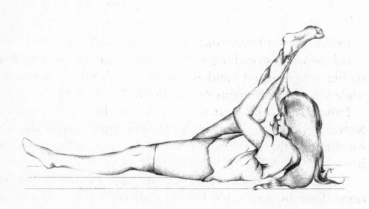

Illustration 16b

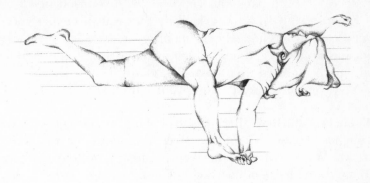

Illustration 16c

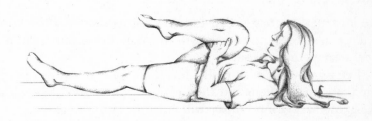

Illustration 16d

Exhale as you lower your back and head down.

Inhale while stretching your leg up toward the ceiling again, sliding your clasped hands up behind it as far as they will go while your head remains on the floor.

Exhale as you lift your torso up in the direction of your leg. Notice if your face is any closer to your knee than it was when you first did this at the beginning of the series of moves. I bet it is!

Inhale as you release your leg up and release your arms to come down by your sides. Flatten your right foot as if you were holding up the ceiling with it.

Keep your foot flat and your leg as straight as possible while you exhale and lower it back down to the starting position.

Relax, and compare your right side with your left side.

Even on your first try, it is likely that you will experience a significant difference. My clients often remark that their right side has stretched and relaxed so much that it feels as if their left side has been lifted up onto a stiff board.

Now, repeat the series using your left leg.

Whenever you have time, spend as long as you can on these stretches. Hold each of the stretching positions for several breaths instead of just one. You've already noticed that even going through them for the hold of one breath has a very noticeable effect on how you feel as well as how much circulation is now getting up into your head and eyes.

VISUAL ADJUSTMENT

Today's new exercise is an intensive stretching that will turn what you've been practicing with the Yoga Eye Stretches into a real near point workout.

Let's get your eyes ready for this workout by increasing circulation into them and then giving them a good loosening. Relaxing background music will enhance everything!

Breathe deeply and yawn often while enjoying a full Facial Massage. Afterward, notice if any areas still feel a little tight. Give them some extra attention!

Your neck can now loosen up, along with your eyes, as you do several minutes of Dot Swings, first with your eyes open and then with them closed.

Now you're ready for the intensive, near-point stretch.

The Mandala Stretch [illustration 17] is a variation of an ancient vision improvement exercise from Tibet. It is similar to the Yoga Eye Stretches, but involves more movements and will further develop your near-point vision.

Get out your eye patch so you can go over the exercise three times, each eye separately and then both together.

Sit or stand at eye level with the Mandala (use this book or

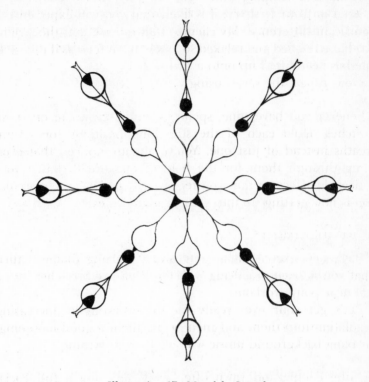

Illustration 17: Mandela Stretch

make a copy of the page), your nose in line with the center and just close enough so that the image is starting to blur. Notice this distance—it will get closer and closer the more you practice this stretch.

Starting from the center, keep your head still and move your eyes smoothly along the outer edges of the design. Breathe and blink.

Once you have visually traced all around the outline of the Mandala in one direction, go back around the other way.

Relax your eyes so they can incorporate the effects with Palming for about twenty breaths. Try some massage afterward to make them even more comfortable.

Look at the printed page. Is it any easier to read?

You can practice this skill virtually anywhere and anytime by visually tracing the outlines of any object. Looking at people is good practice too, but small things near you are the best training for your reading ability.

TODAY

- Be aware of times you're letting stress waste your energy, and choose more positive trains of thought.
- Develop your breath capacity with Full Yoga Lifting Breaths.
- Stretch, yawn, and curl your spine up and down.
- A set of Leg Lifts will revitalize you after your workday is done.
- Use your Fusion String.
- Practice the Mandala Stretch or visually trace the outline of objects close to you.

DAY THIRTEEN

Changing the destructive things you say to yourself when you experience the setbacks that life deals all of us is the central skill of optimism.

Martin Seligman, Ph.D.
Learned Optimism

ATTITUDE ADJUSTMENT

Martin Seligman has been studying optimists and pessimists for more than twenty-five years, and his eye-opening findings are backed up by a concrete method for putting our minds to work for us instead of against us. Unless you lead a totally blissful and healthy life, *Learned Optimism* should be high on your reading list.

Included in the book is a forty-eight-item questionnaire to test your own optimism, which is revealed through your "explanatory style." This is the habitual way in which we explain negative events. Many of us are far more pessimistic than we realize, and it insidiously strangles our efforts to achieve optimal health, success, and fulfillment.

Our explanatory style, whether it's pessimistic or optimistic, can be summed up in three words: personal, permanent, and pervasive. When pessimists think about bad events in their lives, they see them as their own fault, fear things won't get any better, and feel that their whole lives are affected. When the same unpleasant events happen to optimists, they don't take all the responsibility, they are certain things will improve, and they don't let it spoil the rest of their lives.

The same formula holds true for the perception of good events, only in reverse. Optimists consider these personal triumphs, expect the trend to continue, and see them as part of life's pattern. Pessimists think they were just lucky, that it probably won't happen again, and that it won't help with other problems.

For example, let's say someone has spent two weeks enthusiastically participating in a new exercise program, maybe one for vision improvement, when he or she suddenly hits a wall of inertia and allows the next week go by without doing anything at all, the pessimist might think, "I've blown it. I'll never be able to get going again. I always do this." The optimist's explanation would be more like, "Oops, I've had a little lapse. I'll just pick up where I left off. This time around will be better."

Conversely, if it's going well, the pessimist would think, "This is a good program. I wonder if I can keep it up. Too bad I can't do other things this well." The optimist would come back with, "I'm great at this. I'll always be great at this. I always do well when I put my mind to it."

Seligman and other researchers attribute a pessimistic attitude to "learned helplessness." This is the feeling that one's best efforts are to no end and that they have no control of a situation. Low confidence and self-esteem create a cycle of low expectations, which becomes self-fulfilling.

So what's the way out of the vicious cycle? Dogged determination and uncompromisingly positive verbal logic! While I have been espousing positive thoughts, I must admit that Seligman is right when he says that they can often have little or no effect on negative thoughts and behaviors. Not, at any rate, if they aren't backed up by a convincing rationale. Platitudes aren't enough, we must systematically engage in "nonnegative" thinking, feeding our belief systems specific information. Basically, we have to talk ourselves into a positive attitude with persistent and irrefutable logic.

Here are the five ways to accomplish this, according to the cognitive therapy approach recommended by Dr. Seligman:

1. Become aware of recurring reaction patterns that are negatively personal, permanent, and pervasive. Look out for words like *always* and *never*.

2. Logically compile evidence to refute the absolute nature of your negative assumptions. If you've done something badly, conjure up memories of things you have been doing well so the whole picture remains balanced.

3. Explain your perceived shortcoming in a less negative way. Telling yourself you are lazy and hopeless when you lapse in your exercise program sets you up for misery. On the other hand, reminding yourself of your successes with it and acknowledging you need a break gives you a hopeful future.

4. Focus on constructive thoughts. If you can't actually change something, choose not to dwell on it. Acknowledge the problem, then shift your thinking to something else.

5. Identify irrational concepts and replace them with more reasonable ones. "Life should be fair" sets you up for constant disappointment, "you have to take the bad with the good" is more realistic and productive.

To become aware of and make positive changes in our explanatory style can be a profound, life-altering experience. Pay careful attention to your habitual explanations of both bad and good occurrences, and see if you can reword them more optimistically.

BREATHING AFFIRMATION

Let today's phrase give your explanatory style a boost. After your relaxing countdown, keep breathing as you:

Inhale: "Constructive language."

Exhale: "Optimistic outlook."

Yawn and stretch as you count yourself back up. Focus only on the ways in which you feel good!

LIFESTYLE ADJUSTMENT

Today we're going to discuss tips about reading, lighting, and computers, so spend at least five minutes with some lifestyle exercises first. You can certainly choose your own favorites, but my suggestion would be:

Yawn; stretch and curl up and down

Take Rocking and then Rolling Breaths

Do the Leg Lift Series

I've already touched on some important points about reading and lighting, but I'll go in to them more while also confronting how to preserve your sight from its great twentieth-century nemesis, the computer. Good old-fashioned reading from paper pages is less complicated to improve upon than reading from a VDT (video display terminal). Still, most of the same principles apply. For the sake of simplicity, however, I'll divide them into separate categories—book reading and computers. Since the lighting requirements for both are generally the same, let's look at this first.

Lighting

The more light the better (but glare is a no-no).

Even light or white clothing causes glare on VDTs

Full-spectrum lights are best (this includes fluorescent lights).

High-intensity (tensor) lights cause eyestrain.

Book Reading

For reading printed matter or computer screens, good ambient light is important. If your reading or work area is brightly lit but the surrounding area is dark, the contrast causes visual strain. The more contrast, the more strain, which is why the tiny book lights for bedtime reading are an especially bad idea.

Besides a well-lit room, there should be extra light directly on the page you are reading, ideally about two feet behind and a foot to the side of you so there is no glare. Floor lamps should generally have higher wattage than table or desk lamps. Floor lamps work best at 150 watts, while 100 watts is fine on a table, and a desk lamp only needs to be 75 watts.

Posture is important so that circulation to your eyes is not impaired. You want your feet flat on the floor (or a support), thighs horizontal, and your back and neck straight. The best position for the page is centered below horizontal eye level and at a slant parallel to the surface of your face.

Circulation will also be cut off to your eyes if you tense around them or anywhere throughout your face, neck, and shoulders. Those great all-purpose vision savers—breathing and blinking—will automatically relax you. When you get to the end of each page, it's an excellent idea to let out a huge exhalation accompanied by a fluttering of your lids in a series of rapid blinks. Then, before you continue reading, take off your glasses and shift your focus quickly in and out, five times, from far to near objects. This will benefit your close as well as distance vision. Prolonged focusing at the near-point is not a natural function of the eyes, and a break from it lessens the strain. Whenever possible, relax your vision by looking at something about twenty feet away, a distance particularly easy on the eyes.

The big exhalation at the end of the page should not, of course, be the only deep breathing you do during your reading. The more expanded your breathing pattern, the more circulation your eyes will receive. Remember that every yawn brings a flood of nutrient-rich, oxygen-filled, sight-enhancing moisture.

Computers

Computers have made a lot of people rich, and eye doctors must be high on the list. A study by the National Institute of Occupational Health and Safety found that 90 percent of

computer users complained of eyestrain. They develop presbyopia quickly and also report headaches, blurred vision, eye
irritation, slowed refocusing ability, altered color perception,
and even double vision. And then there's the whole question of
the impact of radiation on health and well-being. What's a body,
or an eye, to do?

Having enough ambient and direct lighting is a first step,
though it is even trickier to keep glare off the screen than off of
printed material. As I noted in the Lighting list, even light-
colored and white clothing reflect back on the screen. So, dress
appropriately, and carefully examine your screen for
reflections.

The screen should also be clean. These things create a static
electrical field which attracts dust like a magnet, and the dust
doesn't just cut down visibility, it also irritates our eyes. This can
be compounded by dry air, which tends to be even more of a
problem in many offices where the humidity is purposefully
kept low in order to safeguard the equipment. The machines are
happy, but our eyes, sinuses, and lungs pay the price. My sources
say that frequent trips outside, sinus moisturizing sprays, and
nasal irrigators are the best defense in these situations.

If you get headaches from computer use, they may be related
to sinus problems, but they're even more likely to be traced to
other sources of eyestrain. Lighting may be the culprit, of
course. If you cannot change it in your workplace, I recommend
buying an antiglare screen for your video display terminal. It's
worth talking to an eye doctor about tinted glasses that coordinate with the color of your screen to compensate for bad
lighting. There's a good chance, however, that you may also be
sitting too far from the screen or wearing reading glasses that
aren't appropriate for the distance at which you are sitting.

The natural convergence of our eyes, the focusing together
on the same target for near work, is between eighteen inches
and twenty-six inches. If you're farther back than your optimal
distance, you're straining your eyes whether you're using reading glasses or not. The glasses themselves may also be causing
headaches, especially if you have bifocals or trifocals. You may

be too close for one lens and too far away for another. Although you still need glasses, this is another subject to discuss with your eye doctor. There are now special "computer glasses" designed to fit the demands of the workplace.

Eyestrain can also be produced by the angle of your screen. If it's above your horizontal eye level, the strain is intense. Straight out in front of you is also a strain. Five inches lower is about right for visual comfort. It's ideal if you can tilt the screen the same way you would a book, a little back at the top, so it's parallel with your face. This feature of the notebook computers is one of many that I like about them.

In addition to their maneuverability, notebook screens have LCD (liquid crystal display) screens which have no radiation at all, and, of course, it's much easier to place them in an advantageous position. When I was shopping for my computer and first laid eyes on what became my laptop (that's what they were called way back then), I felt my eyes, neck, and shoulders spontaneously relax. Make one of these little guys your choice, if at all possible.

No matter what type of computer you're using, apply the same rules for posture as you would when reading a book. Now and then, to maintain balanced vision, it's also an excellent idea to shift any printed material you may be using from one side of your computer to the other. And, of course, breathe, blink, yawn, and shift your focus in and out every few minutes.

VISUAL ADJUSTMENT

Let's keep on working out your lenses so they can do their part in the act of reading. This is, in fact, quite a vigorous workout. I expect you're visual system is ready for this, but if you develop eyestrain, slow down or stop and do something more relaxing.

It's eye patch and ball time again. We'll use them first for a hearty round of String Fusion.

Do the same routine you learned on Day Eleven:

Slide one eye at a time up and down the string several times. B and B! (That's breathe and blink, not bed and breakfast.)

Then, use both eyes together, seeing the optical illusion of the two strings crossing as you slide your eyes from knot to knot. Measure where your blur area starts by the number of knots in front of your nose. This number will shrink with practice.

Give your eyes a rest by Palming for at least ten slow deep breaths. Add some massage if they're not fully rested.

Resume bouncing and patching as you flex your lenses in and out with the Near and Far Charts [illustration 18]. This is more hard work, but well worth the effort.

Put your enlarged copy of the Far Chart on a well-lit wall at eye level. Stand far enough back from it so that you can see it clearly. Along with your gentle bouncing or leg balancing, it's also a good time for music, something with a steady rhythmic beat, or even a metronome.

As with String Fusion, do everything first with one eye, then the other, then both together.

Hold your Near Chart in one hand close enough to your face so that the letters are just slightly blurred. As you work your way through the card, you may see these letters come in more clearly, even on the first try.

Start by looking at the first letter of the Far Chart. Take a good look at it. Memorize it. Inhale.

Exhale as you shift your focus to the same letter on the Near Chart.

Inhale as you look out to and quickly study the second letter.

Exhale as you look to this letter on the Near Chart.

Continue in this way all the way through the chart.

When you have finished all three rounds, palm for at least twenty long breaths, then relax into the darkness. Let it feel like your whole body, including your eyes, is breathing.

How has this workout affected your vision right now? If you still feel any strain, massage around your eyes or palm some more.

Where can you place an extra chart or two so that you can practice limbering your lenses in spare moments? Perhaps on office, living room, bedroom, kitchen, or even bathroom walls?

EYES
LOVE
RELAXING

EYES
LOVE
RELAXING

Illustration 18: Near and Far Charts

A number of my clients have also created their own versions of the charts, making a reduced copy of favorite drawings or photos and shifting back and forth between each detail. Another handy way to practice is to hold your watch a little closer than you can read it clearly and shift back and forth, one number at a time, between it and a wall clock.

TODAY

- Explain anything unpleasant that happens without making it personal, permanent, or pervasive.
- Assess the normal lighting when you read or use the computer.
- Pay attention to your reading posture and habits.
- Play with the Near and Far Charts.
- Stretch with the Leg Lift Series.
- Try the Dot Swings to relax after Near-and-Far or String Fusion work.
- Drink a glass of water while out in the sunshine.

DAY FOURTEEN

> Habit with him was all the test of truth, "It must be right: I've done it from my youth."
>
> George Crabbe
> *The Borough*

ATTITUDE ADJUSTMENT

Review time again! You're officially halfway through the Totally Timeless Program now. How long has it taken you to get this far? If it's been two weeks, great! If it's been two months, that's great too! Time is not the issue, except, of course, when we waste it on negative or nonproductive thoughts, attitudes, and beliefs and the actions (or lack thereof) that they produce.

If your original beliefs and attitudes toward restoring vitality to your vision and successful aging weren't as positive as possible, have you felt any shift in them since you began the program? Should the smattering of information and ideas we've covered so far not be enough to lift your expectations, there's more to come, but it would also be helpful to explore as many of the books I've mentioned as possible. It's just a matter of finding the right trigger to jump start positive thoughts and the internal well-being chemicals they'll release.

Keep in mind that self-defeating thought patterns and behaviors are our habits and not our essence. The most persistent and negative ones come loaded with the adrenaline rush of the survival response—not fun, but stimulating, and downright addictive. Trying to just stamp them out is difficult, if not impossible, because only a void is left, and it's our nature to fill a void. If we don't come up with a substitute that is equally or more engaging, we stay with what we know.

This natural tendency to keep the status quo is called homeostasis. It applies to our visual as well as physical, mental, and emotional habits. Trying to change abruptly disrupts our natural rhythms, but gradual adjustments keep us comfortable while the balance tips in favor of the satisfaction of new habits. "Habit," as Mark Twain said, "is habit and not to be flung out of the window, but coaxed downstairs a step at a time."

A great deal of research indicates that it takes about three weeks for new habits to settle in. It's often during the third week that the old habits make a last-ditch effort to hold on. If this coming week has had elements of this for you, know it's natural and use your patient persistence—and a sense of humor! Going over the Attitude Adjustments for this second week is a good way to keep your progress on track.

As you read through them, go over each affirmation several times while taking slow deep breaths.

1. "Gerontophobia is ingrained in all of us, including the elderly."
   Inhaling: "Aging youthfully."
   Exhaling: "Seeing more clearly."

2. "As long as new perceptions continue to enter your brain,

your body can respond in new ways. There is no secret of youth more powerful."
Inhaling: "New perceptions."
Exhaling: "Younger vision."

3. "A powerful agent is the right word. Whenever we come upon one of those intensely right words the resulting effect is physical as well as spiritual, and electrically prompt."
Inhaling and exhaling: The affirmation you created on Day Ten.

4. "Every good thought you think is contributing its share to the ultimate result of your life."
Inhaling: "Good thoughts."
Exhaling: "Good vision."

5. "How efficiently you use your 'stress energy' determines your vitality and your rate of aging. The more efficiently you use this energy, the greater your vitality and the slower your rate of aging—and the better you feel."
Inhaling: "Clear purpose."
Exhaling: "Clear vision."

6. "Changing the destructive things you say to yourself when you experience the setbacks that life deals all of us is one of the central skills of optimism."
Inhaling: "Constructive language."
Exhaling: "Optimistic outlook."

BREATHING AFFIRMATION

Choose one from the above list that will reinforce a change of habit you'd like to continue making. As you relax during the countdown, notice any ways in which this feels different from a week ago. Yawn and stretch after your count back up.

LIFESTYLE ADJUSTMENT

How are the suggested lifestyle habits and exercises coming along? Just as with ideas and thought patterns, the trick for integration of anything new is to be gradual and consistent, yet easygoing and forgiving of any backsliding. Otherwise we end up in the same syndrome as the dieters who eat one cookie, declare their diet ruined, and finish off the rest of the box. Whether in the guise of laziness or outright rebellion, the old habits will try to reassert their control. They especially prey on any and all of our feelings of unworthiness. Each time we fail at self-improvement, it's further proof that we don't deserve our own good care and attention.

Take it from one who knows, the harder we are on ourselves about our temporary failures and setbacks, the more they grow into permanent fixtures. Backhanded compliments are part of the same phenomenon. We give ourselves some credit (I drank six glasses of water today), only to remind ourselves of what else we didn't do (but it should have been eight, and I never yawned once). Be on the lookout for these traps!

Think back on all the positive steps toward a healthier lifestyle that you've made in the last two weeks. See each as a positive move forward, regardless of any lapses or transgressions. Every glass of water, bit of healthy food, vision walk in the sunshine, and improvement in your reading posture and lighting counts as a forward move. The same goes for each lifestyle exercise you've performed.

Every yawn, stretch, abdominal breath, Facial Massage, and Rocking Breath you did during the first week as well as this one has increased circulation into your eyes and whole body. Each has contributed to slowing down, if not already reversing, your aging process, and the effects are not taken away by those you didn't do. Tell that to the nag in your head that represents the entrenched habits the next time it whines at you.

In spite of protests by the status quo, I would expect that the gradual adjustments are starting to have noticeable results. Are you more limber than you were two weeks ago? Has your breathing become any more open and deep? Can you see the results of increased circulation in your face? Can you see more clearly immediately after the exercises and massaging this week than during the first?

Have you felt (and seen) the added benefits of the new

exercises, activities, and information this week? Have vision walks, and general visual awareness, added depth and richness to what you see all around you? Which exercises have been the easiest and which have been the most challenging? Let's go over all the exercises in a review session that I hope you'll find to be a great ten-to fifteen-minute holistic workout. As you'll see, I've mixed those from the first and second week together in what I think is an excellent progressive order. If a different one seems better to you, go for it!

Stretch, yawn, and curl up and down three times. Swing your neck loose slightly during your last time hanging over from the waist.

Sit down and give your face a nice massage. What areas need it the most? Afterward, feel the glow of circulation.

Continue with a set of gentle Neck Stretches. Feel the warmth of your relaxed muscles.

Be aware of your breathing. Open it up with five Full Yoga Lifting Breaths. Ah!

Lie down and take a few moments to notice how your breathing, back, and legs feel now.

Open your breathing more and loosen your lower back with some Rocking Breaths.

Add more stretching by moving into a series of Rolling Breaths.

Finally, do the Leg Lift Series. After stretching the first side, pause to compare it to the other one before continuing.

Relax and savor the results. Stay aware of them when you're up and around again.

How much more limber are you than you were two weeks ago? Was this layout of exercises as effective for waking up or refreshing yourself? Perhaps it can gradually integrate into your lifestyle!

VISUAL ADJUSTMENT

How are your habits of vision coming along? Do you find yourself noticing more about your visual surroundings? Is it more comfortable to be outside without sunglasses? Are you remembering to blink more frequently? And breath, especially when you're under any visual strain?

What about your expectations each time you look at near-point print? Are you remembering to give your eyes a chance to work on their own before resorting to glasses? Is a weaker prescription possible yet? It is likely that a reduced strength will now get you by under good lighting conditions.

The rule of thumb is to use the weakest possible prescription without crossing the line into visual stress. As your vision improves you may find it useful to keep an assortment of different strength glasses for various lighting and reading situations. Your purse or the glove compartment of your car is a good place for the strongest pair. This way they'll be handy when you find yourself in one of those dimly lit restaurants that always seem to have menus with the tiniest possible print.

Even if you're not using a weaker prescription yet, check the distance at which you can read print the most clearly with and without glasses, and compare it to last week and to your starting point. For many pairs of eyes, depending on how long you've been wearing the glasses and how strong they are, this is still very early to see significant changes. But congratulate yourself for all forward steps!

Do you associate any forward steps with any particular exercises from either the first or second week? Consider your experiences with each of the new ones, including the results from doing certain ones "on the ball" (or trampoline, or on one foot at a time). Read through the list before starting on these review week lessons, and compare your initial session to later ones.

If your eyes tire easily during the strenuous accommodation and fusion work, don't push them. Take a break and palm or massage before continuing. Should any of them be too much for you, just stay with the more comfortable ones. Always alter the program to fit your personal needs.

This weeks exercises alone wouldn't provide enough relaxation and gentle loosening as we want, so I've blended in earlier ones for a better all-around review session.

Check your vision before you start. Play some mood enhancing background music!

Begin with three to five minutes of the Hot and Cold Treatment to bring as much circulation into your eyes as possible. (If you need an alternative activity, try Sunning, including its variations of Flashing and the Sun Sandwich.)

Get on the ball, and patch one eye. As you bounce gently, shift your focus from an extended index finger to a red object in the room. Do this with a series of red objects, shifting in and out, letting your visual attention be instinctively drawn to each one.

Change the patch to your other eye, and repeat the process with blue objects in the room.

Move on to String Fusion. Keep right on bouncing, and slide your focus up and down the string, knot to knot, five times. Breathe and blink!

Palm for five long breaths, or as long as you need to. Top this off with some massaging of your forehead, eyebrows, and around your eyes.

Next is the Mandala Stretch. Be close enough to the diagram so the black lines are just starting to blur. Use both eyes together as you follow the line around the design. B and B! Go back around the other way.

Rest your eyes by looking as far into the distance as possible. Take a series of three deep breaths. On each long exhalation, let your eyelids flutter in continuous soft blinks.

Palm for at least three breaths.

On to the Near and Far Charts. Bounce on the ball and use your patch, going back and forth through the charts using each eye separately and then both together. Good!

You have a choice for your final relaxation: either another Hot and Cold Treatment or Palming for about three minutes, followed by a Facial Massage wherever you feel it needed most. If you like the Hot and Cold Treatment, you may find it especially good before and after exercises.

How is your reading ability now? Was this session about right for your eyes at this point? Which exercises and activities are your favorites? Remember, "The best exercises for you are the ones you will do." Don't stall your progress by struggling with anything you find difficult or not to your liking. Do what works for you.

TODAY

- Which affirmations play through your mind? Which might be helpful to counteract any negative thinking?
- Notice how you see and use your eyes compared to two weeks ago.
- Do what you most enjoy that brings circulation into your face and eyes.
- Take a Vision Walk.
- See how many brief moments you can find to direct your relaxed face and closed eyes into the sunshine.
- Give your eyes some Yoga Eye Stretches.

DAY FIFTEEN

If I'd known I was gonna live this long, I'd have taken better care of myself.

Eubie Blake, age one hundred

ATTITUDE ADJUSTMENT

This quip by Eubie Blake became famous when he turned 100, but he began saying it in his relative youth. I know because I witnessed it in person when he was a mere eighty-eight. I was sitting next to him on the piano bench in my father's living room, entranced by the length, strength, and nimbleness of his fingers. He was playing "I'm Just Wild About Harry" while telling the story of originally writing it in waltz time, and he made this same little joke about his age as he stepped up the tempo into the lively one we all associate with this song.

It is a classic of its era in its own right, but the song is also historic in that it was one of the numbers from *Shuffle Along,* Broadway's first black musical. My grandfather was a co-owner of the theater, somewhat involved in the production, and prevailed upon Eubie to work with his would-be songwriter son. The result was a minor radio hit, the launching of my father's career as a songwriter, and the beginning of a friendship and occasional working partnership that lasted nearly fifty years.

It was not my impression that Eubie was ever really a major health reprobate, but he certainly hadn't expended a lot of energy worrying about his health. My father was the one who ate and drank copiously and smoked four packs of unfiltered cigarettes a day. Still, he was always healthy and lived to see eighty-five. Both of these men were kept healthy primarily by their attitudes rather than their lifestyles.

I think their relative life spans make an excellent case for research findings on longevity. For example, Eubie Blake's extra fifteen years of life can be explained by the results of a study by psychologist Bernice Neugarten at the University of Chicago. She found that the most important factor in healthy aging to be "life satisfaction." The following ingredients were found to be the most crucial to true satisfaction.

Enjoyment of daily activities
Optimism
A positive and worthwhile self-image
Feeling there is meaning to one's life
Satisfactory achievement of major goals

Those who live the longest also tend to have a good marriage and happy family lives, low alcohol consumption, and continuous growth in their creativity and careers. Eubie scored far higher on all these counts, perhaps accounting for his longer life span. But considering that my father never had his Broadway show or great acclaim, stopped working at seventy, lived alone, drank heavily, and still lived to be eighty-five, his optimism and enjoyment of life carried him a long way indeed.

In *The Pleasure Prescription,* Dr. Paul Pearsall lists "Twenty

Happy Findings About Health Risks," drawn from research studies that indicate that long life accompanies relaxed attitudes rather than "health terrorism." When all the vital statistics about the things we worry about most are added up, from salt, cancer, and stress to cholesterol, exercise, and diet, it's worry itself that's the most destructive factor.

It would seem that the best prescription for longevity is Arthur Rubenstein's "What good are vitamins? Eat a lobster, eat a pound of caviar—live!" After all, he lived to be ninety-five.

However, here comes the voice of the militant moderate again. Attitude is supreme, but there are physical realities. They usually catch up with us when there's a disparity of balance between mind and body. My father's vision was a good example of this, for in spite of his carefree, upbeat attitude, he was not only presbyopic but also developed both cataracts and macular degeneration. He was not a worrier, but something had to pay the price for all that excessive smoking, drinking, and eating.

Having put all this emphasis on the importance of not obsessing over health matters, in the Lifestyle Adjustment I'm about to turn right around and give you more information than you may want to know about herbs and other vision enhancing substances. They're good for you, they provide a lot of nutritional support to your visual needs, but any you decide to take should be washed down with an equal dose of attitudinal optimism.

BREATHING AFFIRMATION

Every time you've practiced breathing your way down into deep relaxation, you've been increasing your skill at it. As you go through the process today, be aware of this. For now, appreciate how ever much you are able to let go of everything else.

Breathe your way down from ten to one. Allow each number to be accompanied by a feeling of release and deeper relaxation.
    For at least ten more whole-body breaths, say:
    Inhale: "Enjoying today."
    Exhale: "Optimistic about tomorrow."

Let the phrases stay with you are you count and breathe your way back up.

Enjoy today! Be optimistic about tomorrow! Why not? Why waste your valuable "stress energy" on what you can't control? If an energy-squandering worry crops up, how about tickling yourself out of it? Try reminding yourself that you don't want to live in a realm where "tomorrow is the today you worried about yesterday." This works for me!

LIFESTYLE ADJUSTMENT

This is an information day, so get some circulation going in your eyes and body with:

Yawns, stretches, and Spinal Curls
Rocking Breaths and Rolling Breaths
A quick Facial Massage

In an ideal world, we would get all the nutrients we need or optimal visual and physical health through the food we eat. Two factors, of course, interfere with this scenario. Even if we assiduously eat the healthiest foods readily available, they are by and large grown in depleted soil and laden with a variety of chemicals. Most of us, however, also don't eat only what's good for us, regardless of media reminders and our own best intentions. Add this to the extra boost we need for the regeneration process, and you've got a good case for supplements.

Certain vitamins, herbs, minerals, and other nutrients are powerful medicine for our eyesight. There are a lot of them, and you must decide which are right for you. I personally take all the supplements you'll see listed here on a quasi-ongoing basis, trusting my intuition to tell me what I need and when. However, I don't think our bodies like a steady intake of pills. At least for many of us, our systems seem to need an occasional break from the work of digesting and assimilating these powerful nutrients. It's wise to pay attention to your digestion and elimination, and balance your intake so that you remain comfortable.

The older you are the more you need these extra boosts to your visual system. However, chances are that the older you are, the more trouble you may have tolerating and assimilating supplements. Following the directions on the labels, spread out your dosages throughout your day and evening, and unless there are specific directions to the contrary, take them with food. These are all available through health food stores and magazines.

Having made this pitch for supplements, I must also say I don't know anyone who has cured presbyopia with them alone. They help, but they're only part of the picture. Here are the best choices to boost your vision:

Vitamins

VITAMIN A   Not crucial for lens functioning, but extremely important for other parts of the eye, night vision, and alleviating dry eyes. Eat those carrots!

VITAMIN B   The whole complex of B vitamins is important to the healthy functioning of the nervous system, which includes the visual system. A deficiency of the Bs is a major cause of light sensitivity and visual fatigue. B2—riboflavin—seems to be of special importance to the lens.

VITAMIN C   Everything in your body and eyes needs lots of it, especially every cell in your lenses. It is even a major defense against cataracts.

VITAMIN E   Just as crucial as C to your lenses. Think of it as a lubricant!

Minerals

CALCIUM   Needed by the muscles of your eyes as well as the bones of your skeleton

MAGNESIUM   Also necessary for healthy eye muscles

CHROMIUM   Very important in the focusing process!

ZINC   A must for the health of your retina and necessary for the assimilation of vitamin A

Other Nutrients

PROTEIN   The cells of our lenses are made of protein. Feed them well!

COENZYME Q-10   This remarkable substance is a biochemical fuel that helps oxygen ignite ATP, the "basic currency of life," so that every cell in our body is energized, including those in the eyes. It is also especially beneficial for normalizing blood pressure, protecting the heart muscles, and fighting gum disease. There are no final results for people yet, but mice given CoQ-10 had twice the life span as those who didn't receive it. The best natural sources are spinach, nuts, whole grains, sardines, and beef, including organ meats.

Herbs

EYEBRIGHT   This is an herb that increases circulation into the eyes. It helps clear vision and bring a sparkle to the eyes. It can also be used as a wash for eye infections.

BILBERRY   A type of blueberry. I have listed it in this section because it is not available as a fruit, only in tea and capsules. In addition to vitamin C and minerals which benefit every part of the eye, bilberry feeds and stimulates a chemical in the retina known as rodopsin, or visual purple. It is this chemical action which gives us our night vision. The power of bilberry to sharpen night vision was first noticed during World War II, when RAF pilots who ate it regularly as jam developed uncannily keen night vision. Night vision tends to decrease with age. My own took a dip, but as with many of my clients, it returned once I added bilberry to my diet.

GINKO BILOBA   The ginko biloba is the most ancient tree on earth. Its parts have been used in the East as healing and rejuvenating agents for thousands of years. It is an all-around fountain-of-youth tonic, especially for eye, ear, and brain function.

CAYENNE PEPPER   Also known as capsium, you can take this in capsule form (often together with garlic) or use it liberally as a seasoning. It's high in vitamin C, great for your digestion, and wonderful for opening your circulation. It's also powerful against colds.

GARLIC   It's good for everything, including the eyes. It opens circulation, has a purifying effect on our bodily fluids (including those in the eyes), and lowers blood pressure. All of this will also help your eyes regain their flexibility and stay healthy.

PYCNOGENOL   Pycnogenol is the trade name for a substance that is extracted primarily from the bark of the French maritime pine and grape seeds. Research has shown it to be as much as twenty times stronger than vitamin C and fifty times stronger than vitamin E as a free-radical scavenger. It both regenerates and strengthens the cells in the lenses of your eyes. It comes labeled as Pycnogenol, Grape Pips, or Grape Seeds.

VISUAL ADJUSTMENT

It's another strong workout for your lenses today, one that you'll be able to do without charts or a string. But before we start the work, loosen up your eyes with a good three minutes of Long Swings to your favorite music. Be sure to keep it playing throughout the session to minimize the chance of eyestrain.

You can do the next exercise sitting or standing, but the best choice of all would be on the ball.

The Finger Shift [illustration 19] will tune up your eyes' ability to work as a coordinated team while getting your lenses back into shape.

All you need for this is your two index fingers. Hold them up directly out in front of your eyes, one at a distance of about one foot and the other at arms length. They must be lined up one behind the other.

Look right through the near finger to the distant one. Notice that you are seeing it through the optical illusion of the first finger splitting into two images.

Now, shift your focus to the finger closer to your face. Keep your gaze on it, but notice that you can now see the other finger as two images in the background.

The object here is to look back and forth between the two fingers, always seeing the other as two. To get the most from the exercise, it's important to keep breathing and blink often.

Shift ten times in and out. Time your change of focus with your breathing, exhaling as you look in to the near finger.

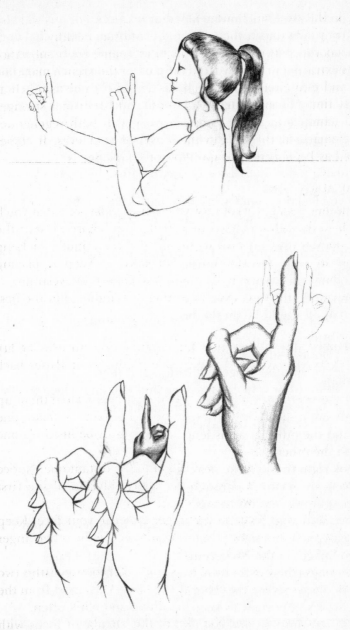

Illustration 19: The Finger Shift

Good. Palm for a minute if you need a rest.

Now comes another set of ten, but with an added challenge.

After you shift in to the near finger, keep your focus on it as you move it in all the way to the tip of your nose and then back out to its original location. Make the whole move on a long exhalation. (This is tough work—don't stick with it if your eyes really complain.)

Then massage your forehead, eyebrows, the bones around your eyes, and anywhere else that calls for attention.

Finally, palm for at least twenty breaths. Think black!

Can you feel how much work your lenses have done? How's your vision without glasses? This is a powerful exercise, so don't overdo it. Too much at once could strain the lens muscles and create a setback instead of a step forward. Small bursts of this activity are ideal.

TODAY

- Notice what you enjoy, what you're optimistic about in the future.
- Consider supplements.
- Play with the Finger Shift now and then.
- Rest afterward with massage and Palming when possible.
- Flex your lenses gently with the Lens Flexor.
- Take in some sun and extra water.
- Yawn and stretch.

DAY SIXTEEN

> How old would you be if you didn't know how old you was?
>
> Satchel Paige
> *How to Stay Young*

ATTITUDE ADJUSTMENT

Even if you're not directly a part of the baby boom generation, it's almost a given that you feel younger than your age, certainly younger than your parents felt at the same age. As I mentioned earlier, psychological age has a verifiable impact on biological age. Lucky us, because never before in human history has there been a time when we have felt so young.

We have every good reason to feel young. Life expectancy has increased dramatically in this century, accounting for two-thirds the total gain since the advent of humankind. In fact, barring cancer and heart disease, women in this country turning fifty from now on can look forward to living into their nineties. If a man has already made it to sixty-five, chances are that he'll see eighty. These are statistics from Gail Sheehy's *New Passages,* and they bode well for our future.

Some twenty years after Sheehy delineated the stages of life in *Passages,* she realized they had already fundamentally changed. Every stage had undergone a shift, but it was the cycles after forty that had radically altered. She sums it up by saying, "Imagine the day you turn forty-five as the infancy of another life...an entirely new concept of the life cycle: a Second Adulthood in middle life."

Every day, more of us over the brink of what used to be considered the start of decline are grasping and integrating bits of this new reality. I agree with Sheehy, however, that the full ramifications of it really haven't hit us yet. Part of our collective consciousness is still operating on the already outmoded timetable of the last generation. Once it sinks in that we really have another forty-five *good* years, we've realized a collective attitude adjustment that will herald a new renaissance.

I recently found myself fascinated by an event that took place on January 23, 1997 (several months from this writing). It was an event in the heavens, the perfect configuration of a six-pointed star created by an exceedingly rare alignment of stars, the sun, and the full moon. The last time this occurred coincided with Europe's entry into the Renaissance. At 17:30 Greenwich Mean Time (GMT), this pattern centered on the first degree of Aquarius. This is considered by many to be the long awaited "dawning of the Age of Aquarius."

Be an optimist now, whether or not you put any stock in the

stars and their influence on us! If it's fate or if it's luck, we're still the group in power as we enter the new millennium. The more we embrace that, the more it enriches as well as rejuvenates us. We have plenty of time, far more than we were ever brought up to expect, to be not only the beneficiaries of this new age but even its leaders. Maybe we'll be the ones to save the world after all.

I've taken the astronomical configuration on January 23, 1997, as a sign, and spent some time in simultaneous meditation with people of like mind all over the globe. As you read this, can you, by chance, remember where you were and how you felt on that day? It was a Thursday. Maybe the events—the Gaia Mind Global Meditation and Prayer, as well as the alignment in the heavens—were in some way noticeable. (You'll see my experience in the last chapter, page 250.)

For whatever reasons, this is an auspicious time. Gail Sheehy breaks down the new Second Adulthood into two stages: the Age of Mastery, forty-five to sixty-five, and the Age of Integrity, sixty-five and over. We're no longer over the hill, we've just hit our stride!

However, only the flexible will find all the changes in store easy to take in stride. In his book *Age Wave,* Ken Dychtwald notes that the social changes that will accompany our expanded life span may have to be fundamental. For example, he projects that we may either never retire or retire several times, and that serial monogamy will become more common than lifelong marriages as our longevity grants us a greater diversity of life cycles. It looks like Art Linkletter was right: "Growing old isn't for sissies."

To achieve Mastery and Integrity as we age may take more conscious effort than ever before. *Successful aging,* perhaps a more appropriate term than *staying young,* is such a long-term prospect that it can be considered a "career choice." Generally, a certain amount of wisdom automatically comes with aging, but getting the most from our longevity will also require ongoing adaptability to continual changes. And, of course, the lenses of our eyes will mirror our inner vision.

BREATHING AFFIRMATION

Now let's put our emphasis on a deep subconscious understanding of the broadened concept of our life span. Let the future and all its opportunities open up to you. Own the fact that you're even younger than you thought you were.

Breathe and count down to a very relaxed ten. Float in the relaxation for a few moments before affirming for the next ten or more breaths (changing the words if you like):

Inhaling: "So much time."

Exhaling: "Just hitting my stride."

Count back up, affirming your energy and vitality. How's your attitude now? "How old would you be if you didn't know how old you was?"

LIFESTYLE ADJUSTMENT

The ideal way to get ready for today's new exercise is with three to five minutes of:

Stretching and yawning while lying on your back
Loosening your hips and lower back with Rocking Breaths
Loosening your shoulders and the rest of your spine with Rolling Breaths

Your position on the floor is perfect for continuing with the Crocodile [illustration 20]. This yoga exercise will loosen and open your shoulders, allowing greater circulation into your eyes as well as the sheer comfort of relaxation in this area.

Before starting, relax on your back and pay attention to how your shoulders feel. Be aware of any tension and the way in which your shoulder blades touch the floor.

Begin lying on your right side. In this position your right knee is slightly bent. Your left knee is more bent, coming over and past your right one. Your arms are stretched out perpendicular to your body, palms together. Your head is also down on the floor.

Stretch your left hand out past your right one. Keep your eyes

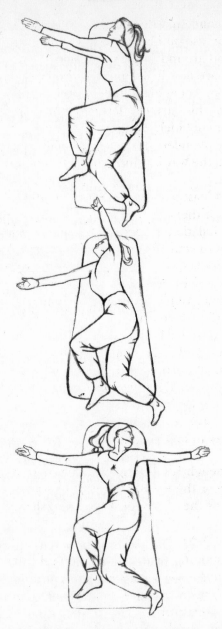

Illustration 20: The Crocodile

on your left hand, and do your best to always keep it in contact with the floor, as you begin slowly sliding it in a giant arc over your head and around to the other side.

Your arms are now in a T position, you're looking at your left hand, and your knees are still bent over to the right.

Relax into this stretch, letting your lower back go and allowing your shoulders to open.

Notice the wonderful stretch through the front of your shoulders and the way in which your left shoulder blade is neatly tucked under.

Hold for at least ten slow and deep breaths, and stretch your eyes along with them.

On your inhalations, slide your gaze out along your arm from your shoulder to your fingertips. As you exhale, slide them back up to your shoulder.

Then bring your left arm back through the arc to your starting position. Watch your hand, keeping it stretched out and on the floor the whole time.

Roll onto your back and relax. Observe the difference between your left and right shoulders. Oh, the poor right one!

Now it gets its turn. Roll onto your left side and repeat the Crocodile with your right arm, including the breathing and eye stretches during the holding period.

After you have returned to the starting position, compare both shoulders to how they felt before you began.

Isn't there a delightful difference? You can, of course, use either the Crocodile or the Rolling Breaths separately, but I think the combination of the two is ideal for a real shoulder treatment.

VISUAL ADJUSTMENT

You have been doing some easy rotations of your shoulder joints and spine, but the word *rotation* is going to take on a whole new dimension in a few minutes. First, get your vision warmed up for this amazing exercise.

Spend about three minutes on the Finger Shift, including bringing your near finger in to your nose.

Relax from this with a brief Facial Massage.

Then, palm for at least ten breaths.

Using the Spiral [illustration 21] is an amazing experience and can dramatically clear your near-point vision. It's not for everyone, however. If you are susceptible to epileptic seizures, *do not* use this exercise. In fact, do not use it if it makes you uncomfortable in any way. Most people thoroughly enjoy the entertaining optical illusion, but a few find it unsettling. If you are one of the latter, do the Dot Swings and use the Near-and-Far Charts while on the ball instead.

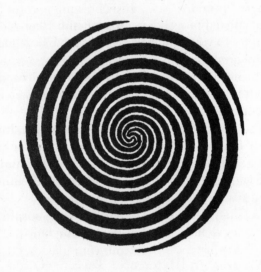

Illustration 21: The Spiral

Take a good look at the Spiral you have photocopied and mounted according to the instructions in this week's Materials List. Is the black good and dark? Part of the effectiveness of this exercise depends on the sharp contrast between the black of the Spiral and the white of the paper. If necessary, make the black darker with a marking pen.

I hope you have located a record player, especially one that has a 45 rpm speed as well as 33 rpm. A portable player is ideal so you can turn it on one side and face it directly. You can lean over one on a horizontal plane, but this puts some strain on your neck and shoulders. Either way, make sure the hole in the center has nice clean and even edges.

If you don't have a turntable, there are several other methods you can use. You can mount the Spiral on a wall with a nail through its center. The hole must be large enough so the Spiral can be spun in circles easily. Whether you sit or stand, place it at eye level. You'll be looking into the center of the Spiral as you use one hand to keep it spinning.

A more practical and portable technique will provide you with a hand-held Spiral. After extensive testing and trails, it was my team of dedicated researchers (Joseph and Jacob Newberry, two of my partner's teenage sons) who determined that the sturdy pin, champagne cork, and cardboard backing for the Spiral are the best materials to use. Pin the Spiral to the rounded end of the cork. You'll be holding the flat end of the cork with one hand and spinning the Spiral with the other as you gaze into its center.

A turntable is best for this because you don't have to turn the Spiral yourself and you're guaranteed smooth continuous movement. The aim is to do this for at least two, but preferably four, minutes. Do the best you can if you're under your own hand power; your skill will increase as you practice.

Before you begin, place this page close by so you'll be able to look at it immediately after finishing your time with the Spiral. Notice how the print looks without your glasses. Of course, keep them off for the exercise.

Stand or sit about sixteen inches from the Spiral, or hold it that far out in front of you.

Gaze at its center as it revolves at 33 rpm or you spin it by hand for two to four minutes in a clockwise direction. Even though you're focusing on the center, be aware of the entire rotating Spiral. Let yourself be drawn into the swirling vortex! It's as if you're opening to a whole new dimension. Breathe, blink occasionally, and watch the center of the Spiral seem to pull in and back from you. Enjoy the illusion!

After the time is up, look at this printed page. What happens? The letters grow larger, clearer, and seem to rise up off the page toward you! The effect may last for about a minute. Look around elsewhere and let the optical illusion entertain you.

How is this going to have a therapeutic effect on your vision? As Dr. Leon Revien, O.D., and Mark Gabor put it in their book *Sports-Vision*, "…with continued practice, a cumulative experience of illusion forms in your memory bank, so that objects can still appear larger in real and practical situations." I would also agree with them, that this is "perhaps the most dramatic exercise for training visual acuity." It is a favorite of many of my clients, both those near- or farsighted, and the drama encourages frequent practice. Hand-held Spirals variety have found their way into many purses and offices.

TODAY

- Doesn't it feel good to know you have so much time, and you've just hit your stride?
- Refresh with either the Crocodile or Rolling Breaths.
- Play with your Spiral.
- Bounce using the Fusion String or the Near and Far Charts.
- Massage your face.
- Fit in a few Yoga Eye Stretches.
- Yawn while curling your spine up and down.

DAY SEVENTEEN

We remember what we understand, we understand only what we pay attention to, we pay attention to what we want. This chain gives us memory. When memory fails, the problem lies in the inability to move along the chain.

Edmund Blair Bolles
Remembering and Forgetting:
An Inquiry Into the Nature of Memory

ATTITUDE ADJUSTMENT

Of all the things we may fear losing as we age, our mind is usually at the top of the list. This fear is one thing we never seem to forget, especially when we've just forgotten something else. Even if you've joined me in banishing from your vernacular such self-sabotaging phrases as "having early Alzheimer's," you may still find yourself worrying about your ever-shrinking brain and the rapid-fire, daily mortality rate of its cells. Old people get forgetful; old people get senile; old people get Alzheimer's. It's inevitable, and it's a damned grim picture.

But it's not true! What we have here is an astounding case of misinformation and misunderstanding! The actual facts about the aging brain are outstandingly encouraging. There's a general impression, for example, that senile dementia and Alzheimer's disease run rampant in the senior population, but less than 15 percent actually suffer these conditions, and many of these instances are considered to have been preventable.

Here's my very favorite fact about the aging brain: it actually grows from mid-life and beyond! You can verify this fact anywhere, but I suggest reading Janet K. Belsky's *Here Tomorrow: Making the Most of Life After Fifty*. Among the encouraging studies she cites is one from Rochester University, which compared the neurons of three groups of dying people, fifty-year-olds, eighty-year-olds, and a group afflicted with dementia averaging about seventy-five years old. To the amazement of the researchers, the neurons in the eighty-year-old brains had more interconnections than the fifty-year-old ones.

It's not the number of brain cells that counts when it comes to memory and learning, it's the connections between them, the neural branches known as dendrites. We may lose some brain cells and the speed of recall with age, but our marvelous three-pound universe compensates for this by developing an average of three million millimeters of dendrites each year between the ages of forty-five and ninety. Our thinking process actually becomes more complex and sophisticated! The stored wisdom and complex reasoning power that we gain more than make up for lost quickness.

So why do we sometimes seem so forgetful and increasingly less intelligent as we age? There are a number of reasons. The modern correlation between speed and intelligence, mistaken as it may be, is certainly a factor. This is compounded by the belief in the whole notion of mental decline as an inevitable result of aging. In fact, studies show that while the young and old score virtually the same on intelligence and memory tests, older people tended to believe they had scored more poorly.

Furthermore, it's likely that all the information we think we're losing was never really put properly into our memory banks in the first place. Memory is a skill as much as a natural trait, and few of us are trained to fully utilize it or keep it sharp. This situation is then worsened by a lack of mental stimulation, lazy or narrow thinking, improper nourishment, depleted oxygen to the brain, and a variety of medications.

If your thinking ever seems fuzzy or your memory spotty, look into any drugs you're taking (especially tranquilizers and high-blood-pressure medications), your diet, physical fitness, water intake, and your attitude toward your current and future brainpower. In addition to improving these basics, we can exercise our brains to increase their agility, stamina, reasoning ability, memory storage, and retrieval skills.

In *Brain Builders! A Lifelong Guide to Sharper Thinking, Better Memory, and an Age-proof Mind,* Richard Leviton presents a "brain building" program in seven sequential steps. Each one is filled with a vast array of exercises and information. This is a big book of activities that could take years to complete, which is great because brain fitness is as much an ongoing project as physical fitness. Consider the seven steps Leviton outlines:

1. Believe your brain—As Leviton writes in *Brain Builders,* "the secret is your attitude." Ahha! Brainpower begins by believing in it.
2. Free your brain—The more you are free from stress, depression, alcohol use, inadequate nutrition, chronic con-stipation, and allergies, the more clearly your brain can function.

3. Get in rhythm with your brain—Discover and harness your own natural cycles of activity and rest.
4. Feed your brain—"Your brain has an outrageous appetite for just about every nutrient known to food science and for about 20 percent of all the oxygen you inhale."
5. Move your brain—Physical exercise pumps more blood and oxygen into your brain.
6. Sound your brain—Our own brain waves are fed by pleasant music and sound frequencies.
7. Exercise your brain—Lastly, we have the mental calisthenics to stretch the brain's limits and keep it on its mental toes.

I have recommended this book to many clients and received back many positive reports. The exercises make for good family entertainment as well as individual use. Either way, use it or lose it—that's the great secret to a quick mind and a sound memory. That, and, of course, a positive attitude. Let's focus on this in today's Breathing Affirmation.

BREATHING AFFIRMATION

Let your mind and body relax as you breathe down from ten to one. For the next ten breaths, focus on:
Inhaling: "Powerful memory."
Exhaling: "Relaxed thinking."

LIFESTYLE ADJUSTMENT

Before we play some brain games, get your body energized as well, taking a total of five minutes for:

Yawning, stretching, and curling up and down
Full Yoga Breaths
Rocking Breaths, a little more vigorously than usual

You're well oxygenated now, so you can get the most out of these mind-sharpening exercises that will also stimulates your visual cortex. Do these in a spirit of lightheartedness. In fact, have a good laugh whenever you get tripped up. One of laughter's many benefits is an increase in circulation which, of course, promotes better vision.

Our first exercise is tongue twisters. Yes, the same game you played countless times as a child. Ah, but with an added twist—the ball! Bounce away as you go through these. The rules of the game are to read quickly and speak out loud—good and loud! No cheating!

Repeat each one three times, each time louder and more rapidly than the previous:

How much hedge would a hedgehog hedge
If a hedgehog could hedge hedge?
Why, he'd hedge as much hedge as a hedgehog could
If a hedgehog could hedge hedge.

A skunk sat on a stump.
The stump thunk the skunk stunk
And the skunk thunk the stump stunk.

Peter Piper picked a peck of pickled peppers.
How many pecks of pickled peppers
Did Peter Piper pick?

She sells seashells down by the seashore.

Betty Baughter bought some butter
But, she said, this butter's bitter.
If I put it in my batter
It will make my batter bitter.
So she bought a bit of better butter,
Put in her bitter batter,
And made her batter better!

How'd you do? Can you think of any more? Go over them out loud too. Use them as warm-ups for vision exercises. Share them with others. Share a good laugh. Spread good cheer, mental agility, and better circulation!

Next, let's read in reverse! This out-of-the-ordinary experience really stimulates brain activity and loosens up your visual system. I have often used this exercise as part of my vision lessons and was pleased to see similar ones in *Brain Builders*! It would be ideal to do this without glasses, but use them if you still really need them. There's no need to read out loud (however, in the beginning you may find it helpful to actually spell each word out loud). The quotations read from left to right, but each word is backward (right to left). Breathe, blink, and keep your shoulders relaxed!

1. "sA gnol sa eno nac erimda dna evol, neht eno si gnuoy reverof." olbaP slasaC

2. "ytirutaM si eht yad uoy evah ruoy tsrif laer hgual ta flesrouy." lehtE eromyrraB

3. "tnemeriteR ta evif-ytxis si suolucidir. nehW I saw evif-ytxis, I llits dah selpmip." egroeG snruB

4. "I eveileb taht eno sah ot eb ytneves erofeb eno si lluf fo egaruoc. ehT gnuoy era syawla detraeh-flah." H. D. ecnerwaL

5. "ehT gniht si ot emoceb a retsam dna ni ruoy dlo ega ot eriuqca eht egaruoc ot od tahw nerdlihc did nehw yeht wenk gnihton." yrneH relliM.

Wow, how's that for shaking loose old patterns! We're not done yet, though. Our next mental workout is based on one by Jean Houston, which appears in its entirety in *The Possible Human*. I often take my workshoppers through the entire twenty to thirty minute experience. If you put the whole script on tape or do it in a group situation, I guarantee you'll find the result worth he effort.

We're going to do a shorter variation here as a visual memory tune-up, but you'll still be able to feel your brain creating new dendrites as you put it through its paces.

Sit comfortably, feet flat on the floor and eyes closed.
Keep your breathing open and easy.
Be aware of the left side of your brain.
Be aware of the right side of your brain.

Go back and forth in this awareness four more times.
On the left side of your brain picture a pink rose.
Let the image vanish.
On the right side of your brain picture a sunflower.
Let it go. As you continue, let go of each image before the
   next one comes up.
On the left see fireworks exploding.
On the right a couple getting married.
On the left a lush jungle.
On the right a snow-covered mountain.
On the left remember the feel of silk.
On the right remember the feel of cold mud.
On the left hear a train coming.
On the right hear church bells.
On the left smell coffee.
On the right smell bread baking.
On the left taste a fresh, juicy peach.
On the right taste chocolate.

You've just balanced and integrated the hemispheres of your
brain, which leads to both clearer thinking and vision. When
trying to remember something, it always helps to activate as
many sense memories as possible.

VISUAL ADJUSTMENT

Today's visual adjustment will bring you a deeper appreciation
of your visual powers as well as greater clarity at near point. It's
also a terrific bit of mental calisthenics, a real memory sharp-
ener. Your lenses need a little workout too, so spend about five
minutes on:

   Bouncing on the ball while shifting your focus from an
      outstretched finger to various colored objects in the room
      (first red, then blue, and so forth).
   Bouncing while using the Near and Far Charts, one eye at a
      time and then both together.
   Palming for ten breaths.

This exercise can be done with any handy photograph or magazine picture. Calendars are often excellent choices. Pick one you have on hand for your introduction to Picture Scanning and Memory. Choose something with lots of colors and details.

The ideal distance at which to hold the picture is at the spot where your vision just starts to blur. You can do this exercise with your glasses on if you need to, but you'll have a greater visual response afterward if you forego them.

Begin by following the outline of the largest object in your picture. As your eyes move around its edges, let your head move along with them a little to the right. As you visually outline this object, be aware of what it is and what colors it contains. Go all the way around in both directions.

Then look for the details within it. Move your head from side to side and let your eyes pick up information like a radar scanner. Mentally name these parts of the whole.

In the same way, move on to each object and significant area of your picture. Work from the largest down to the smallest, taking note of all the interesting colors and details.

When you have taken a good look at everything, close your eyes. Now comes the real fun.

Describe *out loud* what you have just seen. As you do, reach up with the index finger of your nondominant hand and draw in the air what you are describing. Name and draw the objects, their colors, their textures, all the details you can remember. Do this no matter how silly it feels. No peeking!

When you have finished, open your eyes and look at the picture again. Notice how any details that you missed seem to jump out at you. Isn't that amazing? Notice also that the picture looks brighter and clearer.

If you missed anything and usually we do), go back over the picture again. Start with the new details that jumped out at you, then briefly go back over the others as well. Again, close your eyes and go through the process of describing out loud while you draw in air. When you're finished, look at the picture again. If there are more things you missed, and if you have the time, keep repeating the process until you have found and remembered all the details.

Can you see the picture more clearly without your glasses than when you began? Does everything seem brighter and more detailed? How about any print near or in the picture?

Whenever you have time, practice this exercise with all your favorite photographs—you'll find things you had forgotten or completely missed. It's also one of my favorite tips for spending time in a doctor's waiting room. In public places you can skip the air drawing and out-loud description, but be sure to remember everything you can about the picture before you look at it again.

TODAY

- Remind yourself that relaxed thinking produces a powerful memory.
- Scan and memorize another picture.
- Give your eyes the Hot and Cold Treatment
- Do the Leg Lift Series.
- Drink a glass of water while Sunning.
- Practice the Finger Shift.
- Loosen your neck while hanging forward from the waist.

DAY EIGHTEEN

> When your attention is in the past or the future, you are in the field of time, creating age.
>
> Deepak Chopra
> *Ageless Body, Timeless Mind*

ATTITUDE ADJUSTMENT

There are near-life as well as near-death experiences. Near-death experiences are generally rare, profound, and life affirming. The survivor's whole attitude toward life is often transformed, and each moment of every day becomes precious. I'd advise us all to go out and have one if it weren't for the rather depressingly high odds against coming back to reap its benefits. We'd best use ordinary experience to rise to the challenge of discovering that:

> Yesterday's the past,
> Tomorrow's the future.
> But today is a gift.
> That's why they call it the present.

Near-life experiences, by contrast, are all too common, limited in scope, life negating, and drain our life force. They happen every time we dwell on the past or worry about the future instead of live in the present. Each one subtly ages us a little bit more, and for the majority of us these are not isolated instances but a way of life. Paying attention to the moment at hand has become a lost lifestyle, and our wandering attention is aging us en masse.

Where are your thoughts when you take a shower, wash the dishes, cook, drive the car, garden, walk the dog, or mow the lawn? These simple moment-to-moment tasks, decisions, and routines, the very ones we usually think of as mindless, are actually the key to a way of thinking and being that is life affirming and rejuvenating. The art of focusing on the present, be it on making love or soup, is called "mindfulness."

Harvard researcher Ellen Langer defines *mindfulness* as a state of mind and body in which we are "alert, in control, and aware of life's possibilities." Among her most impressive data of the effects of mindfulness on the aging process is a study she conducted at a nursing home. Instead of having everything done and decided for them, as was usually the case, the subjects were given more responsibilities in daily life and taught mental techniques to stay focused on the present moment.

After three years, this group was compared to the other patients. During this time, the mortality rate of the nursing home population was generally 33 percent, but for the subjects of the study it was only 7 percent. And increased longevity was not the only result. In this and similar studies by Langer, mindfulness produced demonstrable improvements in depression, self-confidence, memory, neural brain growth, and health, including hearing and *eyesight*.

Jon Kabat-Zinn, Ph.D., the founder and director of the Stress Reduction Clinic at the University of Massachusetts Medical Center, defines mindfulness as a "moment-to-moment awareness. It is cultivated by purposefully paying attention to things we ordinarily never give a moment's thought to. It is a systematic approach to developing new kinds of control and wisdom in our lives, based on our inner capacities for relaxation, paying attention, awareness, and insight."

Even chronic and acute pain are alleviated when we focus on them mindfully. Dr. Kabat-Zinn, author of *Full Catastrophe Living* and *Wherever You Go, There You Are,* has trained thousands of people to use breathing, meditation, and relaxation techniques to enhance the quality of their lives. Pain may not go away, but to face and cope with it provides far more real comfort than fearing or avoiding it. In fact, to accept that pain is a part of life is a major step toward wholeness as well as health.

We have erroneously been led to believe that pain is an enemy to be stamped out or avoided at all costs. My partner, Jim Newberry, has observed in his twenty years as a bodyworker that people are "obsessed with the pervasive pursuit of a pain-free life." Like Kabat-Zinn, Jim sees his job as not to remove people's pain but to teach them to see it as an ally to be listened to and learned from. Until we're dead, he points out, pain is our own built-in biofeedback mechanism, reporting that something's out of balance, and bearing a message on how to get back on track. If we don't listen, we don't get the message.

If our attention is on whatever is happening in the immediate present, whether pleasurable, painful, or mundane, it can take on meaningful dimensions. Even washing the dishes can become a fascinating sensory interplay of water, bubbles, and touch. What's more, whenever our minds and bodies are interacting together in the moment, they're functioning optimally. Balanced, focused harmony is their most natural state, and this equilibrium has a rejuvenating biochemical effect. By contrast, splitting our attention takes more effort and uses up rather than rebuilds energy.

Of course, we have to consider the past and plan for the future, but these are activities that also benefit from our whole, rather than divided, attention. One of the most challenging activities I ask of people (including myself) is to think and plan only at specific quiet times. When we can do this, we not only conserve and build energy, we generally find that this kind of thinking doesn't deserve any more time.

"Life is what is happening while you are making other plans," is the way John Lennon put it. Ram Dass said, "Be here now." Seeing that the present is all we ever really have makes for real-life rather than near-life experiences.

The ordinary, once we look at it, is extraordinary. When we stop to smell the roses and the coffee, eat without distractions, explore a new route to work, or take a Vision Walk, we're opening to life's real possibilities and slowing down the aging process. Not only that, we best achieve our goals when we fully focus on each step along the way. This concept applies to virtually everything, but a perfect case in point are the exercises in this program. The more your intention is to enjoy them and give them your full attention during your practice, the more you'll be creating youth instead of age.

If you've had any trouble with your attention wandering during the exercises, today's Lifestyle Adjustment is just the thing for you. It's another variation on one from Jean Houston's *The Possible Human,* and there's no way you can do it without being mindful! But first, let's give your attitude its daily adjustment.

BREATHING AFFIRMATION

Really keep your attention only on what you feel as you breathe on your way down from ten to one. Once you've savored the relaxation for a few moments, keep feeling your whole body breathe for ten more breaths while you affirm:

Inhaling: "Living in the present."

Exhaling: "Trusting in the future."

Tell yourself how alert and focused you are as you breathe and count your way back up. Stretch, yawn, enjoy a sense of well-being!

LIFESTYLE ADJUSTMENT

Practice mindfulness perhaps even more consciously than before as you warm up for about five minutes with:

Stretching and yawning while lying down
Rolling Breaths
The Crocodile

Staying totally focused on what you're doing is the only way this next exercise will work. You'll often be moving physically, but this is really a brain game. Through it you'll integrate both hemispheres of your brain, which will produce a heightened sense of body awareness. You may also find that wherever your creative tendencies lie, they will be stimulated during this process. Meanwhile, circulation and energy will flood your brain cells, including those in your eyes, as you engage in this totally out-of-the-ordinary experience.

I call this exercise Kinesthetic Swings. The term *kinesthetic* comes from the Greek words *kinema* (motion) and *esthesia* (sensing). Our kinesthetic awareness is the way in which we sense ourselves in relationship to our environment. The more in touch with this we become the more we develop mind-and-body harmony and increased physical comfort.

If you happen to be myopic as well as presbyopic, you may find this exercise quite challenging at first. Nearsighted people often have limited body awareness, and they generally carry extra mental and visual tension patterns which may initially resist change. This usually manifests itself as a queasy or dizzy sensation. If this happens to you, relax with slow deep breaths and then pick up where you left off.

In workshops where I see that a significant percentage of the group needs this kind of work, I spend a lot of time with kinesthetic exercises. Some, like those you'll be doing today, are of my own invention, but I also rely heavily on many in Jean Houston's *The Possible Human: A Course in Enhancing Your Physical, Mental, and Creative Abilities*. I highly recommend it for thoroughly entertaining ways to keep your body and mind tuned up and integrated. If you have any problems with your balance or are at all accident prone, this type of work can make a world of difference.

Before we begin, stand up and take a short stroll around your room. Look at things around you but keep your main focus on your body. Notice how you feel in your body, how your feet make contact with the floor and how your arms hang. Be aware of your spine and posture.

Let's begin sitting down with both feet on the floor. Close your eyes and focus your attention on your neck.

As slowly as possible, while still maintaining a smooth movement, turn your head to the right. Feel exactly what's happening in all the muscles involved. Study every aspect of the sensation.

When your head and neck have turned as far as they'll comfortably go, continue studying the sensations as you turn your head back to the center, continue the movement all the way to the left, and finally come back to the center.

Next, keep your head still, but imagine that you are going through the whole motion again. Remember and reexperience the same sensations in your neck and head that you had while physically turning them. Take your time, imagining the complete turn to the right, back to the center, left, and center again.

Now comes the fun part.

In the same slow motion, turn your head to the right while imagining you are turning it to the left. Feel the sensation just as clearly in your imaginary head and neck as in your real ones.

Then bring your imaginary and real head back to the center, let them cross each other and continue on to the other side. Stay with this for five or six turns left and right. Breathe!

Good! Now let's try it standing up. We're going to do Long Swings in the same way.

Close your eyes again. First make a complete swing to the

right, back to the center, to the left, and back to the center. Do it as slowly as possible without losing your fluid movement. Feel what's happening throughout your entire body. Repeat until you have noticed and experienced the sensations everywhere, from your feet to the top of your head. Then keep your body still while you imagine it swinging from side to side. Remember and reexperience how this feels in every part of your body. Do this until you have a really good sense of it.

Finally, swing your body in one direction and your imaginary one the opposite way. Immerse yourself in this experience for at least three minutes. Breathe!

Now take another walk around the room. In what ways do you feel different? Do you notice how your feet touch the floor? Your posture? How's your general body awareness? Your vision?

With your total attention on what you were doing, you were living in the present moment and creating vitality instead of age. Practice this kinesthetic imagery as often as possible. You'll get an extra bonus if you apply it to skills you enjoy and would like to improve. For example, it's a great way to improve a golf swing or a dance step, as well as the Rolling Breaths, Yoga Eye Stretches, and many other exercises in this program.

VISUAL ADJUSTMENT

There's a skill coming up that will be the beginning of your reading retraining, but first some preparation:

> Three to five minutes of the Hot and Cold Treatment.
> Several minutes of Long Swings while watching your index fingernail as you move it in and out. B and B!
> Bounce on the ball while your eyes seek out a series of five different colors.

Visual stress and strain, resulting from the aging process or the way we use our eyes or the glasses we wear, interferes with our natural reading skills. One of these is "tracking," the movement of the eyes from target to target. This should be smooth, but it becomes irregular when there's visual tension. By following the black lines of the Maze [illustration 22] with your eyes you'll be retraining them to move fluidly again.

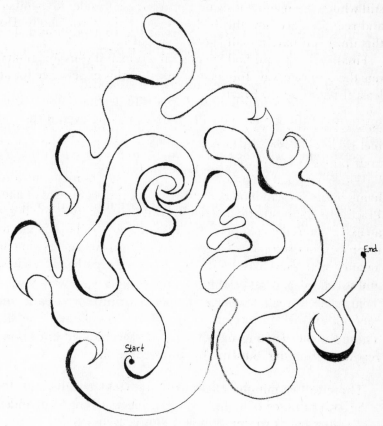

Illustration 22: The Maze

Put the three copies you have made of the Maze (see the Materials List) either on a desk (or table) or on the wall at eye level (you can sit or stand). Line them up so the largest is on the left, then the middle-size one, and the smallest is on the right. Be far enough away so you can see the lines on the biggest one clearly.

Background music can be very helpful here. Choose something with a good strong beat so you can move your eyes along with it.

Begin with the largest Maze. Start at the first point and slide your eyes from there along the line to the next one, and then to the next. That's all there is to it. Follow the line all the way to the end, aware of each point as you cross it. B and B!

Then do the same thing with the middle chart. Your visual memory of the larger one will guide you along even if the line isn't completely clear.

Next, repeat with the smallest chart. You've been over the line twice now; trust your eyes to know the way!

Good.

Now, repeat the whole process, but start at the end point and follow the line back to the starting point.

Excellent!

Enjoy a stretch and a yawn.

Each time you practice this, you're working your way toward being able to read smaller and smaller print more clearly and smoothly. Working with any of the Maze sizes alone is fine, but doing the three in a row gives the exercise an added dimension.

TODAY

- How does it feel to live in the present and trust in the future?
- Do some more Kinesthetic Swings.
- Use the Fusion String or the Near and Far Charts.
- Bounce on the ball while talking on the phone or watching TV.
- Treat your whole body to the Leg Lift Series.
- Get out in the sunshine!
- You can do Full Yoga Lifting Breaths while sitting in the car or watching TV.

DAY NINETEEN

> I won't be old till my feet hurt, and they only hurt
> when I don't let 'em dance enough, so I'll keep right
> on dancing.
>
> Bill "Bojangles" Robinson

ATTITUDE ADJUSTMENT

In Norman Cousins's *Anatomy of an Illness,* there is a chapter
entitled "Creativity and Longevity." In it, he describes meetings
with Pablo Casals and Albert Schweitzer when both were in their
nineties, along with the rejuvenating effect of their love of music
and the playing of it. We don't need to be creative at a master
level to gain benefits, we need only lose ourselves in the
passionate involvement of whatever it may be that entrances us.
Whenever we do something we love, the energy we tap into is
more powerful than science's arsenal of drugs.

Casals's last years personify this fact. Afflicted with emphy-
sema and rheumatoid arthritis, stooped and barely able to walk,
his hands swollen and seemingly crippled, he underwent a
miraculous transformation every time he sat down at the cello or
piano. His back became erect, his breathing opened, and his
fingers unfurled and played with the speed and grace of a young
virtuoso. Cousins relates his own reaction:

> Twice in one day I had seen the miracle. A man almost ninety,
> beset with the infirmities of old age, was able to cast off his
> afflictions, at least temporarily, because he knew he had
> something of overriding importance to do. There was no
> mystery about the way it worked, for it happened every day.
> Creativity for Pablo Casals was the source of his own cor-
> tisone. It is doubtful if any anti-inflammatory medication he
> would have taken would be as powerful or as safe as the
> substances produced by the interaction of his mind and body.

The more we choose to spend time on favorite activities that
challenge us and require skills, the greater the brain-boosting,

age-reversing benefits—within reason, of course. For example, there's a certain time at which the physical, fluid joys of tai chi or aikido begin to make a lot more sense than the thrills of karate.

Some people already know what they thrive on, but many of us have suppressed our needs and inclinations while working to support ourselves and families. A lot of people start to tell me that they have no driving interests and that it's too late to start looking for them. I cut them off pretty fast with my barrage of facts, figures, catalogs for local schools, brochures of organizations, reading lists, and inspirational stories and quotations.

I often quote a point well made by George Leonard in *The Life We Are Given*, which he coauthored with Michael Murphy. He says, "Whatever your age, your upbringing, or your education, what you are made of is mostly unused potential."

Leonard, not only a leader in the Human Potential Movement but also the man who gave it its name, truly knows from where he speaks. He took up the regular practice of aikido well after his passage into middle age and received his first-degree black belt in 1976 after he had entered his sixties. In 1992, he earned his fourth-degree black belt.

The Life We Are Given centers around our need for an ongoing discipline and the benefits of dedicated long-term practice. Michael Murphy is the cofounder and director of the Esalen Institute in Big Sur, California, and George Leonard has always been an integral member of this leading center for personal, spiritual and social growth. After many years of trial and error, they learned that while short bursts of experience could be quite intense, they didn't have lasting depth and effect. It was consistency and perseverance that had the big payoffs; the quick fix was an illusion.

Leonard created Leonard Energy Training, a synthesis of aikido and other disciplines, to expand the rigors of martial arts with other transformative practices. To date, more than fifty thousand people have been introduced to this holistic approach to mind-and-body fitness. Together, Leonard and Murphy introduced an ongoing program through Esalen called Integral

Transformative Practice, which has had a profound impact on its participants.

Their book is a guideline for practice of this overall mind, body, and spirit "path that never ends." I use elements of it with my yoga classes and vision groups, and a number of people have reported finding their whole program a wonderful structure for ongoing development. The majority of those who have stuck with it also use Leonards's excellent video *The Tao of Practice*.

Check out stores and catalogs for videos! Many of us can't get to a class, but technology can now bring the class to us. You may find one program that's perfect for you or a variety that you can alternate between. I have scores of audio as well as videotapes I use myself and loan to clients so they can decide which is best for them.

Whether they go through regular routines at home or in classes, people who cultivate ongoing challenging activities excel in their vision work as well as their general health and attitude. Disciplines like yoga, tai chi, *Qi gong*, and Integral Transformative Practice are popular choices, but so are many less esoteric practices and creative outlets. Tap dancing, ballet, western line dancing, belly dancing, singing, golf, tennis, and playing the piano or other musical instruments are just some of the ways to discover the "transformative power of long-term practice."

The key to staying with something is to remember that it's the journey and not the destination that's important. How much you accomplish is not the point, it's the awareness of always being in process. This endows each repetition of the same thing with the potential for new discovery and learning. As George Leonard says, "In the master's secret mirror, there is an image of the newest student in the class, eager for knowledge, willing to play the fool."

BREATHING AFFIRMATION

Before you feel your whole body breathe and count your way from ten down to one, take a moment to reflect on what changes, if any, you've noticed in your life due to the regular practice of this exercise and the others in this program.

Once you're fully relaxed, let your next ten breaths affirm:
Inhaling: "Regular practice."
Exhaling: "Ongoing growth."
Fully energize as you breathe back up. Stretch and yawn
before you move on to reading about other possible options for
keeping limber and fit in mind and body.

LIFESTYLE ADJUSTMENT

We have another information section for the new Lifestyle
Adjustment, so enjoy a thorough stretching session first. If you
can give it ten minutes, you'll feel wonderful. As you practice the
exercises, place more emphasis on enjoying them than doing
them right. Keep in mind pianist Wanda Landowska's maxim: "I
never practice, I always play."

Yawn while stretching, hanging, and curling up and down.
Do Rolling Breaths
Do the Leg Lift Series
Do the Crocodile

Of all the vision improvement exercises that I teach and practice
myself, the ones I will mention today are my favorites. They are
also the ones usually preferred by my students. I included them
in this section because they shouldn't be limited to the development of your vision. The topic is "fun and games," and should be
a part of everyone's lifestyle.

When I travel to workshops I take a huge suitcase that I call
my bag of tricks. It is filled with brightly colored balls of all sizes,
a variety of rackets, and a huge selection of childrens' toys and
games. My favorite store on earth is Toys "R" Us.

Before I get into some of the best toys and games, let me first
stress the "fun" issue. The whole concept of playing is just as
important as the visual stimulation of the games. There is really
only one rule that governs this concept as I use it here:
noncompetition. On the visual level, once competition enters a
game it creates tension, which interferes with the whole visual
response system. On the human level, competition means there

will be a loser as well as a winner. To be the loser is not fun, and fun is what fosters the good feelings which have healing properties.

Think of *play* as different than *sport*. Play is cooperation, whereas sport is competition. Play is the childlike enjoyment of an activity for its own sake; sport involves winning as its primary goal. Playing is great for the vision. Ordinarily competitive ball-and-racket sports become vision and fun enhancers if you simply play without glasses and don't keep score.

Visually, the object is to always keep your eyes on the ball. Tennis, badminton, and Ping-Pong are wonderful. If you don't have a partner, you can actually do even more for your near-point vision. Hold a racket in each hand and hit the ball back and forth. See how many variations on this you can invent. For instance, hit the ball in the air twice with each racket before changing hands or bounce it up and down using the racket in your nondominant hand. Try doing this while balancing first on one foot and then on the other. Patch an eye every now and then.

Ping-Pong is especially good for your vision. Again, use your eyes so that your lenses get a workout, always keeping your eyes on the ball. Don't play for points, just see how long you can keep the ball in play. Use your patch and your nondominant hand at times. There are no dead balls—hit them when they don't bounce on the table, or after they bounce on the floor. Play with a paddle in each hand.

Ping-Pong is my second all-time favorite vision racket game. My true love is what I call Zenminton. I often spend entire vision lessons with my students playing this game in my backyard. It is the transformation of badminton into a noncompetitive physical and visual delight. The object is to keep the birdie flying as long as possible through an endless variety of variations on the basic badminton strokes. Also, it is played to music, from *Chariots of Fire* to Strauss waltzes.

If you and I were playing Zenminton, we'd almost dance to the music, swirling in circles, lunging dramatically, and leaping with glee. We'd see how slowly and how high we could make the birdie fly, watching it soar all the way in and out from our rackets. While cooperating to keep the birdie in the air, we'd play with nondominant hands, both hands, no hands (well, not really), and wearing eye patches. A high kick in the air while hitting. A quick spin after each hit. You get the idea! The aim is not just to have fun but to free ourselves from habitual patterns. Remember, new perceptions keeps us young.

Even if you can't get set up for Ping-Pong or Zenminton, you can surely play catch with some little balls. Toy stores carry soft ones in a myriad of eye-catching colors. (I always knew those day-glo colors would be good for something!) If you do not have a partner, just toss the ball from one hand to another, bounce it, use the patch, or balance on one leg.

All manner of children's toys and games are great for your vision—marbles, jacks, Hacky Sack, anything that catches your fancy when you explore toy departments. Your eyes will be drawn to items that offer them a chance to play with the changing of focal distances. I won't try to describe the all-time favorite of my clients, but I will tell you it's name. Be on the look out for the Zoom Ball. You'll know what I mean as soon as you see it. (Try Toys "R" Us) If you can find children to play these games with, I guarantee your vision will get yet another boost.

Some party favors are also good vision toys, especially the kind that unroll when you blow into them. These are terrific for your near focusing (even when they also make noises). Get a pack in bright colors, and give one five to ten blows while you watch it without glasses. The little hand-held mazes where you roll the ball from one end to the other are also great for hand-eye coordination as well as visual stimulation. They're handy to keep in a purse or desk drawer for small bursts of vision play.

Do you have any games on hand? If not, plan to go to a toy store or even the toy section of a department store today and see what you can find.

VISUAL ADJUSTMENT

Get out your eye patch again, and we'll jump right into something new for your eyes. The Infinity Stretch [illustration 23] is great as a warm-up exercise, but it stands on its own merits

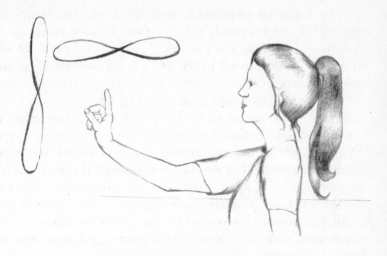

Illustration 23: Infinity Stretch

too. It will flex your lenses, tone up the ciliary as well as extraocular muscles, promote hand-and-eye coordination, develop smooth eye movement, and even balance the hemispheres of your brain. When combined with music, it can help you shift into a desired mood. Play something slow and sweet, and you'll relax. Play something upbeat, and you'll get a real pick-me-up.

Stand comfortably with your weight evenly balanced on both feet.

With your left eye patched, stretch your right arm out in front of you with your thumb up, centered directly between your eyes.

Keep your head still and watch your thumb as you draw a small infinity sign in the air. Draw several in both directions. Breathe and blink!

Keep going, gradually making the symbols bigger and bigger, until your arm is moving at its full range. Then work your way back toward the center, making each symbol smaller than the one before it.

Next, make them gradually larger again, but with an added twist—quite literally. Let your thumb draw the symbols parallel to the ground, as if on a flat surface in front of you. This way you'll be moving your thumb toward and then away from you, giving your lenses more to do. Go from small to large and back again.

Good! Now change hands and eyes and repeat the whole process.

Wonderful! Do it once more, this time with both eyes. Use one arm for awhile and then the other. Let your whole body sway and move to the music.

Now sit down, close your eyes, and feel your lenses moving along with your cupped hands for ten breaths of the Lens Flexor.

Next, put this flexibility to good use with ten Finger Shifts, including watching your near finger move in toward and out from your nose. Exhale whenever your focus shifts in close to you.

Finally, relax into the soothing darkness as you palm for at least ten slow breaths. How about topping it off by massaging your forehead, eyebrows, and the bones around your eyes?

How do your eyes feel? How's your reading ability?

Brief snatches of the Infinity Stretch are one of your many tools for quick visual tune-ups. Many of my clients find reading easier if they warm up visually with these stretches, followed by about a minute of Dot Swings. Try this combo!

TODAY

- Remember that practice as play brings greater growth.
- Can you get to a toy store?
- How often can you slip in a few Infinity Stretches?
- How about some Full Yoga Lifting Breaths? They're a great way to pass the time while in the car, or on train or bus.
- Practice the Finger Shift, on the ball if possible.
- Enjoy a full Facial Massage.
- Hang over from the waist and yawn...and yawn.

DAY TWENTY

> I am saying something as basic as breath: time is life.
> Use it or lose it. Seize it as if you have every right to it,
> like air, take it in, hold it, expand it, shape it to your
> dreams or it will gallop out of control and disappear.
>
>   Letty Cottin Pogrebin
>   *Getting Over Getting Older*

ATTITUDE ADJUSTMENT

Have you heard this one?

An elderly woman emerges from the first Sunday church service she has attended in many months. She tries to slip by the minister unnoticed as he mingles with the parishioners, but he sees her and corners her.

Gently chiding her for her absence, he reminds her, "You know, you are at that stage of life when it is time to think more about why you are here."

"Oh, Reverend," she exclaims, "you are so right. And I am already doing that! I walk into the kitchen, and I think, 'why am I here?' I walk into the bedroom, and think, 'why am I here?' I even open cupboards and think, 'why am I here?'"

A derogatory age joke! But it's funny because this is something we all do. In fact, we've been doing it all our lives. Kids do it constantly. So do adults of all ages. We just think we do it more as we get older. When our thoughts are scattered all over the place, it's easy to lose track of one even while our bodies continue to pursue it.

The joke is also effective because it touches on a serious subject: Why *are* we here? It's a big question, and laughing at it releases some of the pressure. It's also a many-faceted question, covering not only the "big picture," but also our purpose at this stage of our lives, and it puts us face-to-face with our mortality.

No matter how much we chase after eternal youth, we're still going to get older and we're still going to die. You, like me, are most likely more than halfway through your life span. Barring a catastrophic illness or accident, during our later years we will not always be in top-notch condition.

How many good years does that leave, and what is to be the purpose of this time? What do we want to accomplish? What are our goals and priorities? How do we want our epitaphs to read?

As noted earlier, if you're between the ages of forty-five and sixty-five, you are in the stage Gail Sheehy defined in *New Passages* as the Age of Mastery, when we move away from proving ourselves and the survival mode and into more relevant priorities of self-development. Then, in our mid-sixties we enter the Age of Integrity, a transition into a time for acceptance, integration, and reconciliation. However, these shifts don't just descend upon us out of nowhere.

An old Chinese proverb says, "Unless we change direction, we are likely to end up where we are headed." In this age, which Sheehy calls our Second Adulthood, our destination is not the same as it is in the first one. The degree of conscious assessments and decisions involved in successful aging essentially makes it a "career choice." The old question, "What do I want to be when I grow up?" is back again.

How do you see yourself in five years? Ten? Twenty? Thirty? Do you have a plan, other than how to survive as comfortably as possible? Not that financial security isn't important, but what about more personal goals? Try thinking about this for a minute from a particular perspective. Play the "What If" game. We'll play it in two parts.

The first is based on the premise: What if you had no inhibitions about your interests and desires, and no limitations to keep you from satisfying them? How would this ideal life play itself out? Let's use the list of indicators of "life satisfaction" most correlated with longevity. Go through the list three times. For each one, project five, then ten, and then twenty years into the future.

1. Pleasure from daily activities—What would be your ideal daily routine?

2. Regarding life as meaningful—What are the beliefs, interests, activities, and relationships that would bring you fulfillment?

3. Achieving major goals—What would you be looking back on, at the time, and in the future, as personal and professional goals?

4. Positive self-image and feelings of worth—How would you look and feel? In what ways are you pleased with and proud of yourself?

5. Optimism—Of course! Project this as your view of your future. What would you be looking forward to doing? Include your death in your ultimate future and whatever you believe follows it.

Part Two: Do the same thing again, with one important difference. Add the word *attainable*. What would be your ideal, yet attainable, future at each juncture?

Hmmm. How do they compare? Do they interweave? How does your ideal attainable future differ from one you'd project if you were in a pessimistic mood? What can you do to create the optimistic scenario?

BREATHING AFFIRMATION

Let go of the future for now, focus on your breathing, and relax your way down from ten to one. For the next round of ten, affirm the following or a phrase of your creation:

Inhaling: "Living in the now."
Exhaling: "Looking forward to the future."

Fill yourself with more and more energy as you breathe and count back up, alert and choosing to be optimistic!

LIFESTYLE ADJUSTMENT

Before we get started with a new self-massage, spend a few minutes loosening up and bringing circulation into your eyes. How about:

Stretching, hanging, and curling up and down.
Doing some Rolling Breaths.

Did you do the Facial Massage yesterday? How often have you chosen to do it during the program? One of our saddest and most detrimental habits is that of not touching ourselves. Whether this begins as religious, social, or familial conditioning, the end result is self-touch deprivation. Our own touch is as healing as someone else's, but we so often neglect this possibility.

The inner conviction that there is something wrong with bringing pleasurable sensations to ourselves crops up all the time in my vision improvement clients. This is especially true when it comes to the self-massages. People are usually enthusiastic when they begin to use them, but soon find themselves "forgetting" to do them. Have you been falling into this trap, or have you integrated the Facial Massage into your daily life?

Not that you shouldn't integrate massage by others into your life as well! This healing art, in all its forms and related bodywork techniques, has finally become mainstream now that scientific studies verify what people have been experiencing for millennia. Whether it's for stress reduction, a specific physical problem or ailment, or pure pleasure, we should all be massaged by ourselves and others on a regular basis.

I feel so strongly about both the physical and emotional benefits of bodywork (I prefer this more all-encompassing word) that it is very often part of my work in both private sessions and workshops, whether for vision improvement or hypnotherapy for virtually any problem. I have some skill at massage and teach a variety of self-massages, but I depend on a highly talented bodyworker, Jim Newberry, to remove the really deeply set kinks and tension patterns.

Everyone of our workshoppers receives a full bodywork session and several focusing specifically on the head, neck, and shoulders from Jim. In private sessions, hypnosis and bodywork are simultaneous, and the results often extraordinary. I am fortunate to be working with a man who is not only skilled but also intuitively endowed as a healer. If you hear of someone with these qualities, make him or her your choice.

There are many good books available on partnered and self-massage. Trust your intuition on which is best for you. My personal recommendation goes to Meir Schneider's *The Handbook of Self-Healing*. It's massage sections are comprehensive, the vision improvement sections are wonderful, and many other areas of healing are also covered.

Massage bodywork isn't just for better circulation and tight muscles. Its therapeutic values are increasingly recognized every day. A recent study at the University of Miami School of Medicine, for example, found it to be the single best treatment for fibromyalgia, a rheumatic disease with a variety of painful symptoms. Problems with joints, bones, nerves, digestion, internal organ function, well-being of all kinds, and stored negative emotions are also released through healing touch. Many beneficial chemicals are released through touch, but caring, human contact is just as important to healing.

Receiving this care from yourself is something you can do right now. So let's get on with the Head, Neck, and Shoulder Massage [illustration 24].

Begin by giving yourself a good Facial Massage. First take a few moments to become aware of this area, as well as how clearly you are able to read print without glasses. Then give a firm but loving massage to your eyebrows, the bones around your eyes, your forehead, your jaws, and the rest of your face.

Does that feel better? Can you see print more clearly without glasses?

Now we're going to take touch a step further with the Head, Neck, and Shoulder Massage. Pay attention to the way your head, neck, and shoulders feel in comparison to your face. Most likely, you'll notice that these areas feel less alive as well as more tense. As you loosen them up, you'll feel better and see even more clearly.

Start with your scalp. Spread your fingers over your head and dig them in enough so that you can begin shaking your scalp loose from your skull. Bit by bit, you'll be moving your fingers over every part of your scalp. Be thorough; don't forget the very top of your head, the area around your ears, and the base of your skull. Loosen and shake in every possible direction. If any

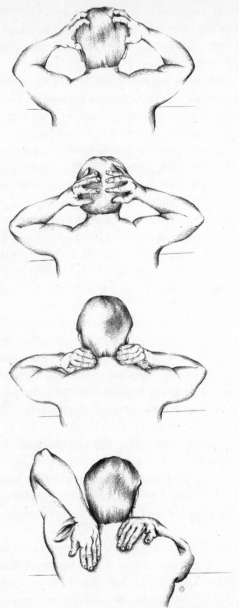

Illustration 24: Head, Neck, and Shoulder Massage

area is tighter or more tender than the others, give it extra attention. Spend about two minutes on your scalp.

Observe the difference. Did you realize that your head could feel so alive and energized? Does this have an effect on how clearly you can read without glasses?

Compare the feelings in your face and head to those in your neck and shoulders. Perhaps you can sense these areas begging for the same attention. They need it!

Start along the base of your skull where your head and neck come together. Spread your hands out over the back of your head, and use your thumbs to massage along this bony ridge. Begin with your thumbs next to one another at the center and work them in opposite directions out to just below your ears. Let your head relax forward and down. Work your thumbs in circular motions as you massage. Give extra attention to any sore spots. These will either be knots of tension of accupressure points, and working them will release more circulation into your eyes. After you have massaged your way out to your ears, work your way back to the center. Then, let your arms relax down as you notice the difference. Compare the areas you have massaged to how you feel down the back of your neck.

To massage your neck, begin at the top. Place the fingers of each hand on either side of your spinal column. Pull out and away from the spine in a hand-over-hand motion, first one way and then the other, and gradually work your way down your neck to your shoulders. Pay special attention to lumps and tight spots. Breath and yawn!

When you reach your shoulders, stop again to rest your arms and hands and to notice the sensations of release and relaxation. Be also aware that your shoulders and upper back want their share of touch.

Start as far down your back as you can reach. Line your fingers up as you did on your neck, digging them in a little on each side of your spine. Again, this will be a hand-over-hand movement. Pull firmly in an outward and upward direction. Stroke all the way over the top of each shoulder. Keep deep breathing and yawning, and work your way up to where you have already massaged your neck.

When you're finished, compare the sensations to before you started. How does everything you've massaged feel now? Are there any places that feel as if they could use a little more massage? If so, give it to them!

How do you feel? How does this page look now without your glasses?

During the day, see when you can indulge in any or all parts of the Head, Neck, and Shoulder Massage. When you don't have time for the whole thing, just be aware of where you need it most. Chances are very good that you'll always see an improvement in your vision after a massage, and the effects are cumulative.

VISUAL ADJUSTMENT

Capitalize on all the circulation you've brought up into your eyes. Start todays workout with a few minutes devoted to:

The Infinity Stretch—separately, then together
The Maze in all three sizes

Your eyes should now be ready for Thumb Fusion, an advanced version of the fusion you've been practicing with the string. If it turns out that you can't do this exercise yet, substitute it with String Fusion. With enough practice, you'll be ready to move on to your thumbs. When you can, it will not only bring in your near-point clarity but also enable you to finally see the 3-D images in those popular *Magic Eye* books.

Like String Fusion, Thumb Fusion [illustration 25] involves the creation of an optical illusion. As your vision converges on a spot in the air in front of your thumbs, you will create a third thumb.

Hold your thumbs out at arms length, almost touching each other. Now cross your eyes and look at a spot in space about halfway out to your thumbs. When you find the right focal

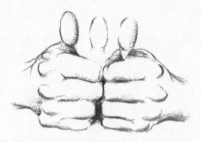

Illustration 25: Thumb Fusion

point, a third thumb will appear between the other two. If you get four thumbs instead of three, this means you're close but not quite there. Breathe and concentrate on pulling the two middle thumbs into one image.

(If you still can't get it, experiment by using two fingers on one hand instead of the thumbs. Make the victory, or peace, sign. This way you can use the index finger of the other hand as a guide for your focal point. Start with it between the two upstretched fingers of the other hand. Keep your focus on this single finger and move it slowly toward your nose. Be aware of the two fingers in the background, but don't shift your focus out to them. A third finger will appear between them when the moving one is about halfway to your nose.

Now the trick is to stay focused on that spot in the air as you lower the single finger down. It may take a little practice, but you'll quickly get the hang of it. Once you can remain focused on the image without the use of the single finger as a guide, you're ready to go on to Thumb Fusion.)

Once you have created the third thumb, you'll begin developing a series of movements while holding onto the image. Be sure to breathe and blink as you do this, and always face your thumbs directly as you move them. (Stop if you feel eyestrain developing.)

Move your thumbs in and out from your face.
Move them back and forth from left to right.

Move them around in big circles: in figure eights; in lazy
eights.

Go back to center now, and hold the image of the third thumb as
you experiment with how far apart you can move your real
thumbs. As you do this, the center image will shrink. In time,
you'll be able to keep the image of a tiny floating thumb in the
center when your hands are up to three feet apart. You need not
go that far for more practice, though. A few inches of separation
will do just fine. Once you can do this, work on maintaining the
image as you go back over the same series of moves that you did
(in and out, circles, etc.) with them together.

It's important to stay visually comfortable when you do
Thumb Fusion. A feeling of having done good hard work is
okay, but real discomfort is not. And it's essential to rest your
eyes afterward.

Indulge in several minutes of Palming, followed by massaging
any area that feels tense.

Since your thumbs are always with you, you can often practice
this in brief spurts. It will both develop your reading ability and
keep it tuned up in the future. Teach it to friends and relatives.
Share it at parties!

TODAY

- Stay focused on the present and expect a good future.
- Notice any face, head, neck, or shoulder tension. Massage
  it!
- Play with Thumb Fusion now and then. Work with your
  Fusion String if you can't get the third thumb.
- Take a Vision Walk.
- Loosen your lenses with the Lens Flexor.
- Yawn and stretch.
- Enjoy the sunshine.

DAY TWENTY-ONE

> Dear God, I pray for patience. And I want it *right now!*
>
> Oren Arnold

ATTITUDE ADJUSTMENT

Three weeks now! How's it going? This is the "normal" time (look for a new definition of "normal" in tomorrow's session for resistance to make its great last stand. Have you transcended the twenty-one-day-struggle and sailed smoothly on through? If so, accolades and champagne! If not, the same! You're still here, and that means, as Star Trek's the Borg would say: resistance is futile. If you have any negative beliefs and expectations about your vision or the whole aging process, they're on the run now. Their days are numbered!

Since we're replacing old habits and beliefs with new and improved ones, the transition may be relatively smooth. If you were despairing about your age at any point, has your attitude improved? Do you feel confident that the rejuvenation of your near-point vision will continue? When you look at your life, do you see opportunities and good times ahead? At the same time, is the present moment as full as possible?

If nonproductive negative thought patterns rear their ugly little heads, trip them up—look at them as good signs! As George Leonard puts it in *The Life We Are Given,* "Your resistance to change is likely to reach its peak when significant change is imminent." I keep trying not to go through these periods of peak resistance in my own ongoing life quests, but they turn up as often as not anyway. I take pride, however, in at least having progressed to an awareness of what's happening. That, combined with using Leonard's quote like a mantra and having a good laugh at myself, has gotten me through some tough moments.

Are there any quotations or affirmations from this week that would be good to keep in mind should any problems in your life or thinking arise? As you go over the list, breathe while repeating each of the Breathing Affirmations several times. Which feels the best to you?

1. "If I'd known I was gonna live this long, I'd have taken better care of myself."
   Inhaling: "Enjoying today."
   Exhaling: "Optimistic about tomorrow."

2. "How old would you be if you didn't know how old you was?"
   Inhaling: "So much time."
   Exhaling: "Just hitting my stride."

3. "We remember what we understand; we understand only what we pay attention to, we pay attention to what we want. This chain gives us memory. When memory fails, the problem lies in the inability to move along the chain."
   Inhaling: "Powerful memory."
   Exhaling: "Relaxed thinking."

4. "When your attention is in the past or the future, you are in the field of time, creating age."
   Inhaling: "Living in the present."
   Exhaling: "Trusting in the future."

5. "I won't be old till my feet hurt, and they only hurt when I don't let 'em dance enough, so I'll keep right on dancing."
   Inhaling: "Regular practice."
   Exhaling: "Ongoing growth."

6. "I am saying something as basic as breath: time is life. Use it or lose it. Seize it as if you have every right to it, like air, take it in, hold it, expand it, shape it to your dreams or it will gallop out of control and disappear."
   Inhaling: "Living in the now."
   Exhaling: "Looking forward to the future."

BREATHING AFFIRMATION

Which one felt the very best, or triggered your own more personally appropriate phrase? Make good use of it, breathe, and repeat it five more times before going on. Yawn and stretch afterward!

LIFESTYLE ADJUSTMENT

The three-week resistance wall strikes down many a diet, smoking cessation, and exercise and self-help program. Therefore, you deserve yet another pat on the back for still being here! Your perseverance is paying off, even if the old habits grumble and complain now and then. Have you soothed your visual system's grumbling with the addition of any herbs or supplements to your diet?

If you haven't been physically active except for the exercises in this program, especially if inactivity has been your pattern for awhile, there's some chance you're getting physical resistance right now. It certainly doesn't happen to everyone, but I became aware of it after teaching yoga for a few years. Around the third week, a fair number of people feel like they're suddenly getting stiffer instead of more flexible. It's that last-ditch effort to maintain homeostasis, the body's clinging to old ways.

This week I purposely introduced only very gentle physical exercises and put the emphasis more on mental loosening. I hope this little ploy was helpful. The tongue twisters, backwards reading, and Kinesthetic Swings are the kinds of activities that free us from habitual mental and physical patterns and facilitate change. If you sense that these mind-and-body integrators and expanders are something you could use more of, take a look into Jean Houston's *The Possible Human* and Richard Leviton's *Brain Builders*. Pursuing games and other activities for the pure enjoyment of play and visual stimulation will also make letting go of old habits easier.

Play! Play a little right now, as part of the lifestyle review. Turn back to pg. 148 and quickly read each tongue twister aloud three times.

Next, read the backward quotations.

Then play with several minutes of Kinesthetic Swings. First do them physically and then mentally. Finally, swing your physical body one way and your mental one in the opposite direction.

Good! Now some stretching, with this week's exercises rounded out with some earlier ones.

Start by lying down. Notice how you feel, the good places as well as any aches and pains.

Enjoy a nice long stretch and big yawns.

Feel a little better already?

Go through the Leg Lift Series, breathing deeply. Compare both sides before doing the second Leg Lift.

Be aware of how you feel through your upper back and shoulders.

Open these areas with the Crocodile. As you hold and relax into the stretch, you can stretch your vision by sliding your gaze up and down your arm.

Now sit up and turn your attention to your face, head, neck, and shoulders.

Yawn and breathe your way through a delicious Facial Massage.

Nice difference?

Now work your way over your head, massaging down your neck and into your shoulders.

Wonderful difference?

How does this page look without your glasses? Expect it to look even better after your Visual Adjustment review session.

VISUAL ADJUSTMENT

Any resistance from your visual system around now? Don't force your eyes to exercise if they rebel against it. There's sometimes a plateau period about this time, when the visual system seems to take a rest while integrating the newly acquired changes. Should this occur, indulge the need and spend a few days (or even weeks) with just the visual activities you find restful and easy. Enjoy Vision Walks, Sunning, Palming, or whatever strikes your fancy. On the other hand, you may very well be effortlessly synthesizing all the adjustments and ready to forge ahead into greater clarity. I'm pulling for the latter!

Whether you're resting or charging forward (or should that be backward, since this is age reversal?), how is your near-point vision compared to three weeks ago? To last week? If it improved and then stabilized or slipped back somewhat, that's generally a sign that gentle exercises and circulation builders like the Hot and Cold Treatment are in order for awhile.

If all is going well and you are stress free, spend as much time as possible on today's review session. If your eyes complain about any of the exercises, substitute something more relaxing. Let's capitalize on the circulation you've brought into your ocular area using the massages. Do you have some rhythmic music to play?

Begin with a minute or two of Finger Shifts. Include the step of watching your finger come toward and back out from the tip of your nose. Breathe and blink!

Palm for a minute, then massage around your eyes, eyebrows, and forehead.

Next, take three or four minutes to play with your Spiral and the illusion of the print rising up toward you afterward. (If you need a substitute, Dot Swings are a good choice.)

Use this enhanced perception for a quick practice at Picture Memory. Use any handy picture, preferably one with colors, details, and some print. Scan around the biggest objects first, and work your way down to the smaller details. Close your eyes. Remember the picture, describe it out loud, and then draw it in the air with your nondominant index finger. Open your eyes and see what you missed. Resolve to practice this important skill more often!

Move on to the Maze. Use both eyes together quickly sliding your eyes along the black line from beginning to end and back again.

Now, the Infinity Stretch. Using both eyes together, watch your thumb tracing the infinity sign out in front of you, on both the horizontal and vertical planes. Breath, blink, and notice how the background zooms by in the opposite direction of your thumb as you watch it.

Relax and palm for five or six breaths. Do you need a little massage around your eyes?

Finally, give Thumb Fusion a try. Breathe, blink, and play with it for awhile. If it just doesn't work yet, play with String Fusion instead.

Now really let your eyes relax. Palm for at least ten to twenty long breaths. Think black. The more it develops, the more your visual system is relaxing. How about a little more massage as a reward for a job well done?

Is the printed page any more clear? So far all we've done is let improved reading clarity appear on its own after the limbering exercises. Starting tomorrow, however, you'll begin putting all this groundwork into actual reading skills.

TODAY

- Let the various affirmations play around in your head. Which comes back most often?
- Give your eyes a chance to read print before putting on glasses.
- Is there somewhere outside with a nice view where you could do a few minutes of Long Swings?
- Count a few colors everywhere you go.
- Memorize another photograph.
- Nourish your eyes with sunshine and water.
- Compare your vision and how you use your eyes now to three weeks ago.

DAY TWENTY-TWO

Joy and fulfillment keep us healthy and extend life.

Deepak Chopra
Ageless Body, Timeless Mind

ATTITUDE ADJUSTMENT

How happy are we? How much joy and fulfillment do we experience in our lives? We want these at the core of our lives, yet we often only flirt with them. Many of us suffer from what Dr. Paul Pearsall calls Delight Deficiency Syndrome. In *The Pleasure Prescription,* he lists ten symptoms of this condition. Are you suffering from any of these:

1. *Chronic fatigue*—tired all the time, and usually not able to sleep well
2. *Constriction*—physical tenseness, most often in shoulder, neck, and head
3. *Chronophobia*—fear of time (there's never enough for what you need to do)
4. *Consumerism*—always wanting more and better
5. *Feeling conflicted*—work and relationships get in the way of each other
6. *Feeling cornered*—dreams unfulfilled, trapped by realities
7. *Being controlling*—if things aren't the way you like them, you feel threatened
8. *Feeling challenged*—always having to prove yourself
9. *Becoming careless*—making mistakes, and more mistakes, even little ones
10. *Being cynical*—looking on the downside or unable to take pleasure in simple activities

Well, I have my ups and downs, How about you? I do very well with my energy level and harmony between my work and personal life, but I have my moments with the other symptoms. However, I must say that I give myself a lot of extra points for catching myself falling into these traps and taking steps to adjust my attitude, even though it's a challenge (symptom number 8!). It helps to remember that the root derivation of the word *perfect* is "finished," which we won't be until we are dead. That takes some of the pressure off.

Look at this list again. Doesn't it seem like the human condition? In fact, except for fatigue, carelessness, and feeling cornered, these qualities are pretty much held up as virtues in our society. They are supposed to spur us on to greater heights. It's normal to feel these things.

Normal. There's an interesting word. There are various ways to define it, but I go with one of the founding fathers of modern psychology, Abraham Maslow. He determined that: "Certainly it seems more and more clear that what we call 'normal' in psychology is really a psychopathology of the average, so undramatic and so widely spread that we don't even notice it."

The "psychopathology of the average," how's that for putting normalcy in its place! Remember this when you read the poem that will be part of your visual adjustment tomorrow; it's a license to greater freedom of self-expression. The trick, of course, is to discover how to break rather than just recognize our self-defeating habits and behaviors. I've found that another list of Paul Pearsall's is helpful in this endeavor. This one is from his book *Super Joy: Learning to Celebrate Everyday Life*. He has developed a new science he calls "joyology." There are twelve principles of joyology:

1. *We come to feel as we behave.* Action creates emotion. Act "as if" you feel good, and the real feeling will follow. Try this: make a big smile and hold it for one minute—you'll see!

2. *We learn more from studying happy, healthy people than we can learn from the exclusive study of the sick and the stressed.* Science is finally realizing this. Do the same thing in real life—learn from and spend time with happy people.

3. *There are an infinite number of states of human consciousness.* Real joy doesn't come without a willingness to allow and move fluidly through the whole range of human emotions.

4. *The brain is not as important as it keeps telling us it is.* It's listening to our hearts and intuitions, and feeling deeper empathy that bring us joy.

5. *The brain is a gland, not a computer.* It floods us with mood-altering chemicals determined by the emotions we feel. "Stress" chemicals age us; "joy" chemicals rejuvenate us.

6. *The brain is first and foremost a health maintenance system.* Its

main function is our short-term survival, but we have to keep reminding it we want long-term joy.

7. *We are not our brain.* Our consciousness far exceeds the confines of our skull.

8. *The brain is too lazy for joy.* Simple survival is easier than a long-term strategy for well-being. Persistence pays!

9. *The best immune system booster is a shot of super joy.* Persistence toward joy pays off in our health, too.

10. *All disease is brain disease.* Consider the idea that human selfishness contributes to society's diseases.

11. *The best drug-testing program is the human brain.* Once our joy chemicals—the psychochemicals known as endorphins—kick in, they are at least as pleasurable as anything mankind has synthesized.

12. *Being healthy isn't enough.* We must add life to years, not just year to life!

To actively seek out the experience of joy is to take risks, bond, communicate more deeply, and live fully in each moment. Our time to do this is getting shorter, yet once we enter into the process we have all the time in the world.

BREATHING AFFIRMATION

Deep relaxation releases endorphins. How deeply can you relax as you breathe and count down from ten to one? For the next ten breaths, affirm:

Inhaling: "I choose"

Exhaling: "Joy and fulfillment."

Let the simple joy of being alive fill you as you count up into refreshed alertness.

LIFESTYLE ADJUSTMENT

The new exercise for today will be done standing up, so get ready by spending a few minutes lying down and warming up with:

Stretching, yawning, and curling up and down at least five times.
Remember that both the upward and downward curls are on
your exhalations.

Rocking Breaths
Rolling Breaths
The Leg Lift Series

The Leg Lifts just stretched most of your back nicely, so let's
expand on this by bringing the stretch up further, into your
shoulders, upper back, and chest. Notice how these areas feel
now. The Chest Expansion [illustration 26] will open and relax
these areas, stretch out your legs, and bring a healthy dose of
circulation into your face and eyes. In fact, I've seen women's
magazines call this a minifacial.

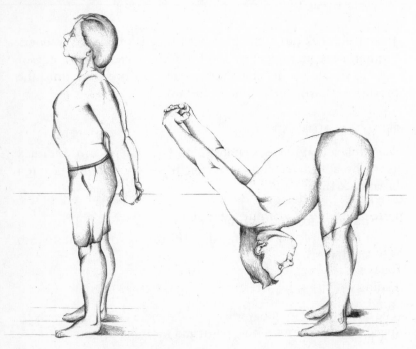

Illustration 26: Chest Expansion

Standing upright, stretch your arms out to your sides, then bring them in front of you with your fingertips together and your palms facing away from you.

Inhale as you bring your arms out and around behind you, and clasp your hands.

Hold this breath as you look up and stretch up toward the ceiling. Squeeze your shoulder blades together gently and downward.

Exhale as you stretch out and then down in front of your legs. Look through your legs rather than at the floor in front of them so that your neck stays relaxed. Bring your arms up as high over your head as possible.

Take three or four easy breaths as you hang over in this position. Feel how everything relaxes a little more into the stretch with each one of your breaths out. Be aware of all the circulation coming up into your face, eyes, and brain.

The next step involves an inhalation, but if you have any tendency toward dizziness when standing up too quickly, leave out this breath until you've practiced awhile.

Inhale and come upright again, taking a little stretch up with your face and again gently squeezing your shoulder blades together.

Let go of the stretch and relax for a few moments with your eyes closed, feeling its effects. Do you have time for another one? Or two?

This is a great energizer even if you're not bothered by tightness through your shoulders. If you get "office back," this is the perfect antidote. Computer users take note!

VISUAL ADJUSTMENT

Today we're going to do some close work in preparation for the reading exercises this week. It's a very effortless exercise, so let's round out the session with a few that are more of a workout. Take a total of at least five minutes, preferably on the ball, for:

A little Sunning.

String Fusion while on the ball.

Thumb Fusion (substitute Near and Far Charts if your eyes
   still aren't quite ready for this), also on the ball.
Relaxing with some massage and Palming

The Picket Fence Swing [illustration 27] is similar to the Dot
Swings but stimulates even more visual movement. Working
with the three drawings in descending size gives your eyes a
nonthreatening reintroduction to relaxing while reading small
print.

The exercise is extremely simple but very effective. Because it
is so repetitive, however, pleasant background music can really
provide an added impetus to keep going. Anything you would
use for Long Swings will be perfect.

Begin with the largest drawing.

Maintaining good posture, hold the page at a comfortable
distance (it's okay if everything is not clear), and remember to
breathe and blink often.

Point your nose and eyes at the end fence post on the left, and
then swing them across the rails of the fence to the post on the
right. Your eyes and head move together, back and forth, in a
steady easy motion.

As you slide from side to side over the rails of the fence,
pretend there's a stick attached to the end of your nose. As a
child you no doubt ran by fences and bounced a stick along the
rails. That's what you're doing now with your nose stick.

Remember the tick-tick-tick sound that the stick and fence
made? Do that now as you run your imaginary stick over the
picture. Out loud! Really! It's fun, and the auditory stimulation
boosts the visual one. You should be able to feel your eyes
vibrating with movement.

As you tick-tick-tick your way to and fro, be aware that as with
the Dot Swings, there is an apparent opposite movement taking
place. As you swing left over the fence, it appears to be moving
to the right, and vice versa.

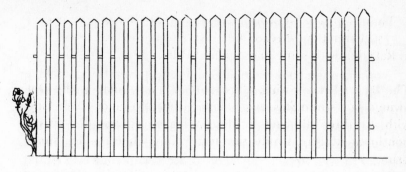

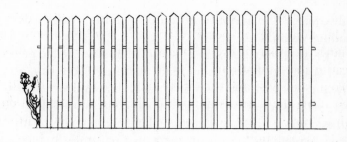

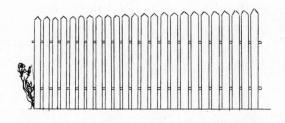

Illustration 27: Picket Fence Swing

After one minute, repeat with the middle fence.

Then the smallest.

Good.

Now, turn the book on its side and repeat everything, making up and down vertical swings over the fence from the top post to the bottom one. Keep the sound going! Blink!

Finally, put the book down. Close your eyes and imagine the page of picket fences suspended in the air about fourteen inches in front of you. Repeat the whole process with your eyes closed but moving your head as you imagine your stick tick-tick-ticking over the fence posts.

Palm for a few long breaths when you're finished. Can you feel your eyes vibrating with energy?

Can you feel the liveliness in your eyes? How does it affect your reading vision?

It's a good idea to make copies of the picket fence page for a quick tune-up before you read anything. You can also use anything with similar rows of lines. Rulers and yardsticks work very well, especially if there's a good contrast of colors. Combs can become quite entertaining. Clients who come to my home for vision lessons leave with their own naturally striped turkey feather, courtesy of the wild ones that roam through the yard. There are lots of possibilities!

TODAY

- Why not choose joy and fulfillment?
- Refresh yourself with the Chest Expansion.
- Tick-tick-tick over real picket fences too!
- Stretch your neck now and then.
- And you eyes with Yoga Eye Stretches.
- Relax with Sunning.
- Yawn between sips of water.

DAY TWENTY-THREE

> Do not take life too seriously. You will never get out of
> it alive.
>
> Elbert Hubbard

ATTITUDE ADJUSTMENT

Psychologists have coined a term to define the opposite of
"*dis*tress"; they call it "*eus*tress." Distress, like anger, grief, fear,
and emotional turmoil, shuts down our immune system. "Eu-
stress," positive emotions and, in particular, hearty laughter,
boost endorphin levels and raise immune system function by
lowering serum cortisol in the blood.

Reader's Digest always reminded us that "laughter is the best
medicine," and we knew this deep down all along. There had
been intermittent studies on the benefits of laughter, but it took
Norman Cousins's 1979 book *Anatomy of an Illness* to rekindle
interest and instigate a landslide of scientific studies to provide
"proof," of laughter's benefit. Researchers stuck in their elec-
trodes, drew blood, measured brain activity, and, yes, feeling
good is definitely good for us. Regular ongoing doses of upbeat
emotion extend life in the long run, and a shot of uproarious
mirth brings an instant physiological lift.

Some of the findings on laughter are really impressive and
can be an enormous boon, especially to the infirm or exercise-
phobic among us. For example, a three-minute raucous guffaw
is as good for us as ten minutes on a rowing machine. The
intestinal stimulation from just one hilarious minute is esti-
mated to have the same effect as two ounces of fiber. All tears
flush toxins from our bodies, but those that accompany hard
laughter wash out two times more than other types of tears. A
really good laugh brings with it thirty-six hours of increased
immune system elevation. The endorphins produced by ten
minutes of belly laughs can bring two hours of pain relief.

Norman Cousins made extensive use of the analgesic effects
of laughter during his 1964 bout with ankylosing spondylitis, a
disease which disintegrates the connective tissue in the spine.

When he found there was no cure for this painful and nearly always fatal disease, he took matters into his own hands. After determining that the pain medications were exacerbating the condition, that vitamin C appeared to be the best treatment, and that positive emotions could boost his immune system, he took action. Deciding that hospitals were depressing, inefficient, unsanitary, coldhearted, and that the appalling quality of the food was enough to kill him, Cousins checked himself out and moved into a hotel room.

Armed with a good attitude and support system, intravenous ascorbic acid, Marx Brothers' films, and *Candid Camera* episodes, he made a miraculous recovery, even though its completion took some years. He had initially enlisted the aid of the comedies solely as mood elevators, but was surprised and ecstatic to discover the pain-killing quality of laughter. After about two hours, when the effects wore off, he cranked up the projector again and commenced guffawing until he was again pain free.

The ability to manipulate our moods, to consciously shift from a bad one to a good one, affects our thinking as well as our health. In *Emotional Intelligence: Why It Can Matter More Than IQ,* Daniel Goleman notes the intellectual benefits of a good mood and hearty laughter. People who can harness their emotions and will themselves into a better mood think more clearly and succeed more easily than those who cannot shake free of anxiety and depression. The complex and flexible thinking process necessary for innovation, problem solving, and creativity is stultified by negativity and anxiety.

Some really good news is that even stepping briefly out of this mental paralysis can produce measurable improvements in thinking ability. For example, a 1991 study titled "The Influence of Positive Affect on Clinical Problem Solving" (don't you love those scientific titles?) showed that creative solutions came far more readily after the subjects watched comedy videos. Breaking out of a cycle of worry and anxiety can be as simple as turning on the TV or having someone tell you a good joke.

Laughing expands and clears the mind, and good moods provoke more of the positive and adventurous decisions that make for richer life experiences. What's more, I've noticed that if the laughing matter pertains directly to the problem at hand, the results can be absolutely transformative.

Bill, a forty-five-year-old trial lawyer and one of my pres-byopic clients, is a perfect example of the transformational power of humor. His reading glasses and mid-life crisis had arrived hand in hand. Twenty years as a prosecuting attorney had left him with a grim opinion of human nature. His dissertations on the "essential evil of man," coupled with six months of Freudian analysis, had his wife on the verge of leaving him. In fact, I wasn't too pleased with him myself, since he kept trying to force clear vision and then had bursts of anger when this strategy failed.

One day after a lesson that included a discussion on the futility of life, I impulsively sent him home with tapes of a talk by Dr. Stanislav Grof, called "The Cosmic Game." In it, Grof, a pioneer of transpersonal psychology, discusses the nature of consciousness and the universe, including the presence of evil. Using a story about the holy man Rama Krishna, he illustrates his point that it takes polar opposites, such as good and evil, to create a whole. A disciple asks the master why there is evil, and after a small pause and with a sly grin he responds, "To thicken the plot."

I had a feeling that Bill might understand this point of view as explained by Grof, who began his career as a rather cynical and highly intellectualized Freudian analyst. I love it when I'm right! Bill "got it." This view, that life is a cosmic game of con-sciousness unfolding and exploring itself in infinite ways, made sense to him. When "It thickens the plot" came along, he literally fell on the floor laughing. As he sat up, his eyes fell on a magazine article he'd been reading about warring religious factions in Bosnia. Then his laughter became tinged with sadness as he wished they could see the larger perspective.

Bill then realized that he was reading the article without his glasses. This was his first visual breakthrough, and I imagine it had as much to do with making new sense of life as well as a good hearty laugh. He made quick progress after that, soon needing glasses only in dim restaurants and similar places. I'm also happy to report that once his attitudes relaxed, his marriage got back on track and his career took on a new light. He also became a confirmed laugher, and swears that watching morning cartoons on TV while dressing is the perfect way to start a day.

Geroge Santayana had it right when he said, "There is no cure for birth and death save to enjoy the interval."

When the brain has lost its healthy sense of humor, it often has to be consciously jump-started back into action. Remember the effect of holding a real smile for a minute? Happiness can bring a smile to our faces, but we can also initiate happiness by smiling. It's a good start!

BREATHING AFFIRMATION

Let a small smile of contentment play on your face as you breathe and relax your way from ten down to one. It can stay there as you affirm for ten more breaths:

Inhaling: "I choose"

Exhaling: "Laughter and joy."

Now, a big smile (crinkle your eyes too!) as you count up and energize.

Ah! Isn't that nice?

LIFESTYLE ADJUSTMENT

Today, how about a thirty-six-hour immune-system boost from three minutes of laughing? First, let's get your chest and breathing opened so you can get maximum benefit from your guffaws. Warm up for five minutes or more with:

Yawning and stretching on the floor
Rolling Breaths
Full Yoga Breaths
The Chest Expansion

Consider yourself an honorary member of Laughing Clubs International (LCI). Yes, there really is such a club, though all the official chapters are in India! After reading about it only recently in a lead story of *Health* magazine entitled "Can You Laugh Your Stress Away?" I immediately incorporated their "exercises" into my yoga and vision classes. We may open the first chapters in the United States. These laughers are really on to something!

Bombay, a city where keeping a sense of humor can be a real challenge, has twenty-eight laughing clubs, thanks to LCI founder Madan Kataria (clearly an enlightened man, since he has a mere forty-one years of life experience). There's no fee. People, usually a group of forty or more, meet in parks and just "stand around in the pink, polluted light of dawn, busting their guts for no apparent reason." After the first fifteen meetings they ran out of good jokes, so they settled on a systematic blend of deep-breathing exercises, loud belly laughs, and others with names like Silent Laughter With Mouth Open, Silent Laughter With Mouth Closed, and Ho-Ho, Ha-Ha. Participants claim better health, lower blood pressure, less stress, weight loss, improved sleep, and a caring support group.

I'm not a stand-up comedian, but in addition to the new Bombay belly laughs, I've long tried to inject humor and laughter into my workshops. It makes for camaraderie and precipitates bursts of visual clarity. One of my standard tools is an audiotape of nothing but forty-five minutes of laughter. It's impossible to resist joining in. When my group has been taking themselves too seriously, I just punch on the tape and get them back into the right mood.

Your mission, and I do hope you choose to accept it, is to look for more ways to bring humor and laughter into your life. There are an infinite variety of ways to do so without a laughing club, but research shows that people in group situations laugh 30 percent more often than when by themselves. Still, there are a lot of great comic movies and TV shows, including cartoons. Jokes can come from books and magazines as well as other people, but it's a great idea just to start sharing jokes with your friends and family. Having a pet never fails to lead to amusing entertainment. Even calamities can bring a smile if you remember, "if this is going to be funny later, then it's funny right now."

Meanwhile, a little laughter right now is in order.

Have you heard the one about the Buddhist monk in front of a hot dog stand in New York City? He looks at the astounding number of choices of toppings and finally says, "Make me one with everything."

Remember what Lily Tomlin says: "The problem is that even if you win the rat race, you're still a rat."

When Zsa Zsa was asked which of the famous Gabor women was really the oldest, she answered, "You'll never get her to admit it, but actually it's Mama."

What does a compulsive shopper have in common with an angry bull? They charge everything!

"He's got the whole world in his pants..."—Often mistakenly heard as the first line to "He's Got the Whole World in His Hands."

Do you know how you can tell if you are a codependent when you die? Someone else's life flashes before your eyes.

Okay, okay, now you see why the Bombay Laughers Club quickly moved on from jokes to pure laughter! You must know some better ones. Can you think of any right now? I think the important thing to remember about getting benefits from jokes is to be forgiving. Laugh at the bad ones too!

Try pure laughter in the style of the Bombay Laughers. If you look in the mirror, I guarantee a big laugh! Do at least thirty seconds each of:

Silent Laughter With Mouth Closed
Silent Laughter With Mouth Open
Some hearty ho-ho-hos
Some he-he-hes
Giggling
A *huge* ha-ha-ha

Finally, remember the classic negative suggestion to try not to think about a pink elephant? Here's one better: *Try not to think about smiling!*

Gotcha! Whenever you need a smile just try *not* to think about it and, poof, you'll have a good one.

VISUAL ADJUSTMENT

In a few minutes you'll be reading something that will bring a smile to your face as you begin learning a technique that will help clear near-point print. Spend at least five minutes getting your eyes ready with:

String Fusion on the ball
Dot Swings
Picket Fence Swings

The first line of the poem printed below (in letters four times larger than the print in the book) became the title for the collection of inspirational pieces on aging, entitled *When I Am an Old Woman I Shall Wear Purple.* The "reading" you will practice with it has nothing to do with how well you can see the black print, so you definitely won't need your glasses.

The object here is to focus on white rather than black. This will get your visual system over its expectation of failure when it comes to reading. As this happens, you'll see the print start to come in more clearly.

Rather than "reading" the poem, you'll be sliding your gaze along the whiteness, under and around the lines of print and words. The idea is to pretend you have a bright white magic marker attached to the end of your nose. With it, you will be highlighting between the lines and then around individual words.

Move your head and eyes together. The first time through the poem just highlight the whiteness between the rows, highlighting from left to right and then back again to the left on each before going to the next.

As you do this, several optical illusions may appear. The lines of print may seem to move in the opposite direction of your

Warning
by Jenny Joseph

When I am an old woman I shall wear
  purple
With a red hat which doesn't go, and doesn't
  suit me.
And I shall spend my pension on brandy
  and summer gloves
And satin sandals, and say we've no money
  for butter.
I shall sit down on the pavement when I'm
  tired
And gobble up samples in shops and press
  alarm bells
And run my stick along public railings
And make up for the sobriety of my youth.
I shall go out in my slippers in the rain
And pick the flowers in other people's
  gardens
And learn to spit.

You can wear terrible shirts and grow more
  fat
And eat three pounds of sausages at a go
Or only bread and pickles for a week
And hoard pens and pencils and beermats
  and things in boxes.

But now we must have clothes that keep us
  dry
And pay our rent and not swear in the street
And set a good example for the children.
We must have friends to dinner and read the
  papers.

But maybe I ought to practice a little now?
So people who know me are not too shocked
  and surprised
When suddenly I am old, and start to wear
  purple.

slide, just as with the Dot Swings and Picket Fence Swings. In addition, the whiteness you're imagining drawing under the lines may actually start to glow brightly. Let it happen! Whether or not you get the glow, you'll still most likely begin seeing print flash in more clearly on the periphery of your vision, even on your first practice. Don't shift your focus to it; keep on sliding by on the whiteness.

The second time you go over the poem, highlight the white all the way around each word. Let your head move freely and play with different directions and highlighting patterns. Again, as you ignore the words themselves, they'll begin to jump out clearly at you when you go by them.

Breathe and blink!

How did your vision respond? You can practice this in brief spurts now and then, like many of our other exercises. The more you see the white, the more you'll see the black.

TODAY

- Laugh at nothing! Laugh at everything!
- Tell someone a joke.
- Have someone tell you a joke.
- Enjoy some Long Swings outdoors.
- Highlight some white before reading.
- Practice the Infinity Stretch.
- Bounce while playing with Near and Far Charts
- Yawn and yawn while hanging over from the waist.

DAY TWENTY-FOUR

Jonathan Livingston Seagull discovered that boredom and fear and anger are the reasons a gull's life is so short, and with these gone from his thought, he lived a fine long life indeed.

Richard Bach
Jonathan Livingston Seagull

ATTITUDE ADJUSTMENT

Jonathan Livingston Seagull was committed to optimal experience; to stretching the limits, and to accomplishing something worthwhile. It was his natural inclination to break away from the constricted mind-set of the flock, but it took hard work and dedication to achieve his goals. The crux of the erstwhile bird's success, however, was not the act of perseverance but, rather, his sheer enjoyment of each challenging flight.

The heroic quest and total involvement of the acrobatic, high-flying gull was manifested in his optimal, or "flow," experiences. Dr. Mihaly Csikszentmihalyi, a University of Chicago professor and a long-time researcher on optimal experience, has found that there's no way of getting around the fact that "To improve life one must improve the quality of experience." When we do this with whole-hearted enjoyment, there simply isn't any room left for anger, fear, boredom, or the miseries of aging.

In *Flow: The Psychology of Optimal Experience*, Csikszentmihalyi makes a distinction between "pleasure" and "enjoyment." He sees pleasure as necessary for contentment and satisfaction, but enjoyment as a source of psychological growth. By his definitions, it is possible to attain pleasure without any effort, such as watching TV, eating, or drinking alcohol. Enjoyment goes beyond passive pleasure in that it is derived through active involvement, concentration, and meeting challenges, such as playing chess, a musical instrument, or a hard-fought tennis match.

Paul Pearsall certainly includes these qualities within his use of the word *pleasure*, but Csikszentmihalyi's emphasizes the stimulation of the brain through complex concepts and tasks. These are a must if we are to enter into flow experiences, which bring not just deeper immediate enjoyment but actually enhance the span as well as quality of our lives. Energy expended when we are absorbed in complex tasks builds, rather than drains, the life force. Intense enjoyment pays back a dividend of brain development that strengthens as well as satisfies.

Csikszentmihalyi's studies have revealed that a truly enjoyable, flow experience has eight possible characteristics. If any or all of these occur, we reap life-enhancing benefits.

THE ELEMENTS OF ENJOYMENT

1. A challenge that takes skill, yet offers the chance of successful completion—This could be anything from rock climbing to solving math problems to reading.
2. Total concentration on the activity—Action and awareness merge, and we are totally absorbed in the experience, whether it's ballet, chess, or the perfect golf swing.
3. Clear goals—The possibilities range from a chess match to a bridge tournament, from gardening to building a house to writing a song or poem.
4. Immediate feedback—We know if we've won or lost the game, whether or not we've made it to the top of the mountain or played the right or wrong note.
5. Effortless but deep involvement—Awareness of everything else drops away because concentration is so intense. The focus could be hiking in nature, a science experiment, a musical piece, or even a holiday during which we truly let go of everyday concerns.
6. A feeling of being in control—This is when there is some risk involved, yet we feel we are exercising control. Surgeons experience this in the operating room, hang gliders in the air, chess players in a series of strategic moves.
7. A loss of self-consciousness—Totally absorbed in a challenging activity with clear-cut goals, we can forget ourselves as well as our problems. It's not a loss of self, but a getting out of one's own way and blending with the experience. This can occur while engaging in anything from playing a musical instrument to fly fishing, dancing, riding a horse, or acting.
8. Altered time perception—Occasionally time seems to stand still, but, more often, it flies by when we are engrossed in the task at hand.

Inherent in all the factors of enjoyment is that the activity is to be indulged in for its own sake. Money, prestige, even winning, are not as important as the activity itself. They may come along with it, but true brain-boosting, youth-preserving enjoyment ensues when rewards are secondary to the experience.

To keep sharp physically and mentally, it pays to discover and explore a variety of avenues of enjoyment. It also pays to examine any activities that you engage in because they are good for you even though you don't enjoy them. The benefits of real enjoyment warrant finding alternatives. Let's say, for example, that you work out regularly on machines at a gym but find this tedious and boring or distract yourself with the TVs often provided. This is not a flow experience. Alternatives to explore could be running outdoors, yoga, the martial arts and related, but more gentle, oriental disciplines like tai chi, or a variety of sports, dance, or even mindful walking.

Mental flow comes in many varieties as well. Now it's time for more and deeper interests, not fewer. It's not too late to study that language you always meant to. In fact, its the perfect time. The more we indulge now in learning anything we enjoy, the greater the extra payoff in health and well-being. Remembering also aids both memory and cognitive skills, making constructing the family history or an autobiographical narrative an activity to consider. The concentration and creativity involved in writing is another bonus.

When we lose ourselves in the creative flow of writing, making music, painting, photography, working with materials such as clay or wood, or any artistic undertaking, we nourish ourselves. Indeed, even eating and sex nourish our whole being if we approach them as art forms. All the senses respond with enjoyment to conscious attention. Our hearing, as well as our soul and mind, is stimulated when we are absorbed in listening to music. Smell, touch, and, of course, vision are enriched when we give them our full attentive appreciation. The more we "flow" the more we grow.

BREATHING AFFIRMATION

How much enjoyment can you experience as you do today's Breathing Affirmation? Concentrate on the pleasure of relaxing and adopting even more positive thought patterns, and you have a flow situation. Breathe down and then affirm for ten more breaths:

Inhaling: "To enjoy"
Exhaling: "Is to live."

Energize with deep breaths as you count up, affirming liveliness and enjoyment.

LIFESTYLE ADJUSTMENT

Let's make it a full massage day. Close your eyes for a moment and focus on how you feel throughout your face, head, neck, and shoulders. How do your eyes feel? When you open them, observe the clarity of the print. Wait till you see the difference in a few minutes! Yawn often as you start off with:

The Head, Neck, and Shoulder Massage
The Facial Massage

Today's addition to your lifestyle is yet another massage, and its power will be increased by visualization. The Chinese Acupressure Massage [illustration 28] has long been used to combat visual fatigue and increase acuity. My clients have found that, when combined with a little imagery, its effects are even more evident.

Spend about four minutes with this massage, one for each point or series of points that you will rub firmly. Soothing background music will help the time go faster and keep you in the right state of mind. Go over the process once just to locate the points, then really do it along with breathing and visualizing.

Use your thumbs to massage the first points. They are located where the bone around your eye curves up into the eyebrow area. You'll find an indentation there, and it will most likely be tender to your touch. You want to develop the sensation the Chinese call a "sour" feeling: a tolerable pain that doesn't cross the line into self-torture. Rub in circular motions and focus on the sensation as well as your abdominal breathing.

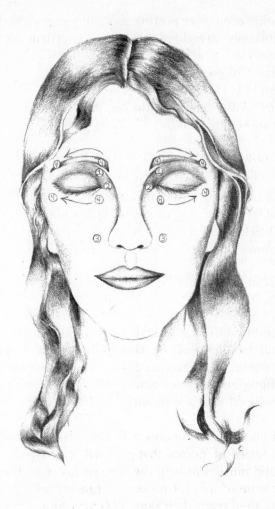

Illustration 28: Acupressure Message

Use a little imagination as you massage. Think of your breath as energy, and give it a color, perhaps seeing it as a white, gold, or blue light. How would it feel as well as look if your breath was flowing from your lungs into your arms, down them, and out through your thumbs into the points you are massaging, and then into the lenses of your eyes? Imagine your lenses glowing with the energy you are sending into them. Stay with this visualization throughout the exercise.

After a minute, move on to the second points. You'll use just one hand to massage both at the same time. These points are just in from the corners of your eyes, and feel like little grains of sand or fatty nodules. Press in and out on them gently—there should be no pain involved here. Breathe and send energy through them to your eyes.

The third points can be a little tricky to locate. They are on the cheekbones where they curve down and under. Take a careful look at the illustration. Most people tend to look for the points too high up. Be sure the top corner of your middle finger is lined up with the bottom edge of your nostril, and that the middle fingers are lying flat against your face as you use them to line up with the points.

Press your index fingers down next to your middle ones. It's the index fingers that are on the points. So, fold your middle fingers under. When you press in with your index fingers, you should find very tender spots, much more tender than even the first one. If it's not especially tender where you are pressing, explore along the bottom edge of your cheekbone for a spot that is. Breathe energy into them and imagine it flowing into your eyes.

The fourth place to massage is a series of points above and below the eyes. The traditional Chinese method is to curl the index fingers and use the big knuckle to stroke across the top bone and then the bottom one in outward movements. You may certainly use this technique if you like it. I, along with many of my clients, feel that this involves too much pulling on the delicate tissues around the eyes. So we use our thumbs on the top bone and index fingers on the bottom ones, rubbing back and forth in the same way you learned for the basic massage around the eye areas.

When you are finished, relax with your eyes still closed. Feel how all these areas, and your eyes, are pulsating with energy. Know that they are energized and flexible with circulation. Appreciate the fact that these points you have stimulated also release healthy energy into your sinuses.

Did the Acupressure Massage have an immediate impact on your vision? This is often the case, but it's still doing valuable work even if you can't see the difference right away. Even when you can't find the time for a full Acupressure Massage, use any part of it you're instinctively drawn to as a mini-energizing session. Every one helps!

VISUAL ADJUSTMENT

This session's new exercise is, like the Maze, important to reading ability but not an advanced skill. If you haven't already seen some substantial improvement in your near-point clarity, the Labyrinth [illustration 29] is an excellent activity to work with often. If, on the other hand, your reading is coming along well, it will become just one of your many tools to use occasionally to keep your skills honed.

Let's weave the Labyrinth into a good all-around visual workout.

Begin with some Sunning, indoors if need be. Let the soothing warmth and light both relax and stimulate your vision for about two minutes.

As you sun, swing your head in every possible direction past it, always aware behind your closed lids that the sun is moving in the opposite direction of your swing.

Let go of your head movement, and do a little Flashing of your fingers back and forth between the light and your lids.

Then, make five Sun Sandwiches.

Next, use your Spiral for two to four minutes. If it's not for you, substitute the Picket Fence Swing. Breathe! Look at print immediately afterward.

Now explore the Labyrinth. You'll be going through it three times, once with each eye patched and then with both together.

Instead of following the black line as you did with the Maze, let your eyes slide along the white space between the lines. Start at the first opening and let your gaze move smoothly along the white path to the end. Breathe and blink!

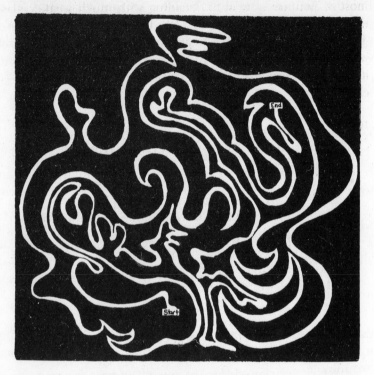

Illustration 29: The Labyrinth

When you get to the end, reverse your direction and follow the white back to the beginning.

Good!

Get on the ball now, and bounce your vision around the room, seeking out colors. Look for reds, yellows, blues, and others.

Keep bouncing gently, and do the Finger Shift for about a minute. Unless it causes discomfort, include the advanced move of watching your near finger come all the way toward your nose between shifts to the distant finger.

Finally, palm again, taking twenty breaths this time. Really relax: let it feel like your eyes and whole body are breathing.

How did this workout affect your reading clarity? I expect that most of you are now either reading with much weaker glasses than when you began or are already free of them completely. The farther you still have to go, the more you need to scan for white and use the Labyrinth. You can, of course, make copies of it for use elsewhere, including reduced sizes for more of a challenge.

TODAY

- What "exercise" do you most enjoy? How can you enjoy it more often?
- Do all or parts of the Acupressure Massage.
- Slide through the Labyrinth again.
- Treat your shoulders to the Chest Expansion, followed by the Crocodile.
- Play with some tongue twisters.
- Play some kind of game involving a ball.
- Highlight white before reading.

DAY TWENTY-FIVE

When we acknowledge the comedy of time, we recover
the power of memory. Like time, memory can be
recovered at any point and brought into the eternal
now. Like time, too, all its strands and forces can be
gathered for the edification of the present. If you have
lost or blocked your memories, chances are you have
also blocked or lost the times of your life.

Jean Houston
The Possible Human

ATTITUDE ADJUSTMENT

The potential of conscious study and thoughtful, creative interpretation of our personal and family history as a flow experience
is abundantly rich. On the surface, it first might seem like a basic
conflict with the whole concept of living in the present, but not
if it's done right. Dwelling on and wallowing around in specific

areas of the past is entirely different than recalling the whole and learning from it.

Our personal history can be a veritable gold mine of insight, introspection, emotional growth, and creative expression as well as straightforward brain function and memory-sharpening exercise. Have you ever tried to go back over your whole life, tracing the significant events, trends, details, and life decisions? It's certainly absorbing and definitely challenging. The gaps are just as important as the vivid recollections, and, boy, oh boy, do most of us have some gaping holes in our memory banks. Filling them in makes us more whole and complex, from our emotional balance to our ongoing growth of neural dentrite.

The most vivid memories from a particular period of time are a good place to start. Recording and interpreting them very often triggers recall of all manner of related details and events we didn't even know we remembered. Bringing out the old photo albums, home movies, and other memorabilia becomes a flow experience when the guiding purpose is a viable product, perhaps a gift to younger generations of your family, and a structured way to make sense of the past. This then continues into the challenges of insightful examination and creative presentation, be it written, audio- or videotaped, or using a combination of media.

Whenever possible, it's valuable and often enlightening and healing to compare your memories with others who were present at the time. Different perspectives provide added details, and sometimes entirely divergent viewpoints of the same occurrence. This can even become an opportunity to clear up misunderstandings, release old wounds, to finally forgive. It's a chance to move beyond nursing old grudges or escaping into lingering fantasies over what was or might have been. It's a time in which the past can expand the present.

We who are only in our fifties, or even younger, can benefit from putting our pasts in perspective just as much as those who have greater distances to review. This isn't just something to do when we think we have all the ends tied up, it's pertinent at any stage of life. Whenever we stop to take a good close look at our history, we have an opportunity to take better control of its future course.

If you've felt like an out-of-control pack rat compulsively storing away bits of the ever-fading past, you're exonerated! If you have been harsh on other family members who do this, repent! Souvenirs, mementos, even all those shoe boxes of unsorted photos, used consciously, are valuable clues to who we are and where we go from here. I don't know about you, but it does me good to get over these recriminations on both accounts. I was hard on my mother for all her hoarding of things whose time had gone by, and then hard on myself for not being able to stop myself from following in her footsteps. Instead, it feels wonderful to see the shed I have jammed with stuff as my own personal historical museum.

In Csikszentimihalyi's chapter, "The Flow of Thought," the section on history as an optimal experience is subtitled "Befriending Clio." In Greek mythology, Clio, "the Proclaimer," was the muse of history. This also happens to have been my mother's name. Of course, I knew the derivation of her name, but when I suddenly saw her lifelong accumulation of memories in the context of her role as historian, it was a gleeful moment of, Ah Ha! So I dedicate this Attitude Adjustment to my mother. Thanks Dr. C!

I only recently came across a large manila envelope of letters my mother had saved. As far as I can tell, it contains every one I wrote to her from the time I left for college until her death ten years later. Whenever I read one, I am invariably flabbergasted by the blank spaces in what I thought was an era firmly etched in my memory. Who were those young men I dated and wrote home about in great detail! What was the field trip to the observatory with my students when I was teaching high school? I knew I had blocked out a few bad memories, but I had no idea so many others fell by the wayside along with them!

Now when consciously recovering the times of my life, I often use an exercise derived from *The Possible Human,* one that is also standard in my vision workshops. After breathing down into relaxation, I recall a series of positive past events. For example, when the Christmas Santa brought me a saddle, my first day of school, my twenty-first birthday, my first day of teaching; my wedding day...my second wedding day...my third wedding day (oh well, live and someday learn!). Then, with memory banks primed for access, I reach for a recollection around the time of the blank space I'm trying to fill in. While remembering as many sensory and emotional details as possible, the whole process of memory expands and forgotten peripheral details, people, and events begin to pop back up. Try this—you're even more interesting than you thought!

The willingness to look at ourselves up close fosters visual as well as emotional clarity. Consider, if you will, my paraphrase of the opening quote from Jean Houston. I have substituted the word *vision* for *memory*. Are they not one in the same?

"When we acknowledge the comedy of time, we recover the power of vision. Like time, vision can be recovered at any point and brought into the eternal now. Like time, all its strands and forces can be gathered for the edification of the present. If you have lost or blocked your vision, chances are you have also blocked or lost the times of your life."

BREATHING AFFIRMATION

You may have some spontaneous past memories during today's Breathing Affirmation. Or you may not. If they surface, follow them if they lead you somewhere that's really valuable right now. If not, let them wait for another time.

Relax. Feel your whole body releasing with each breath out from ten down to one. Then, use the next ten to affirm:

Inhaling: "Remembering the past."

Exhaling: "Clearing the present."

Breathe deeply on your way up into a refreshed and alert present!

LIFESTYLE ADJUSTMENT

Let's focus on the flexibility of your spine today, stretching and rotating it in a number of directions. The yoga saying, "You are as young as your spine is supple," is so true. Before you begin with our series of exercises, be aware of how your back feels now. Move it around a little and get a really clear sense of it "before" comparing it to how it will feel in just a few minutes.

Before the new exercise of the day, we'll start with five or six minutes of the following:

Yawn noisily and stretch lazily and luxuriously.

Curl your spine up and down at least four times. Move on your exhalations.

Lie down for a few minutes of Rolling Breaths. Breathe deeply as you roll smoothly and continuously. At the end of each exhalation, quickly dart your gaze up and down your out-stretched arm.

Move on to the Leg Lift Series, still breathing and moving in smooth coordination. Compare sides before you stretch the second one. Enjoy the total effect afterward.

Sit up and compare your back, indeed, your whole body, to how it felt before these stretches and spinal looseners.

A delightful improvement, I'm sure, but wait till you discover how much more spinal mobility you really have! You'll be able to literally see as well as feel a marked difference after just a few repetitions of the Spinal Twist [illustration 30].

Sit with both knees down and to the right and your feet to the left. Lean back on your right hand for support, and bring your left hand out in front of you, the back of it facing you. Keep your eyes on this hand throughout the exercise.

Inhale. While exhaling, smoothly and slowly swivel your torso and arm around to the right. Twist as far around as you comfortably can.

Hold the twist as you inhale, and look past the ends of your fingers to see what they are lined up with in the distance. You are measuring how far you have rotated your spine. Mentally mark this point—a place on the wall, furniture, or whatever.

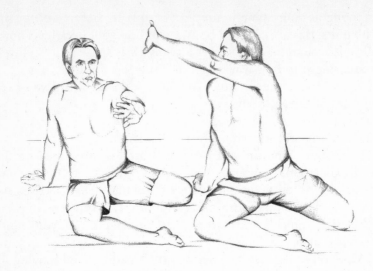

Illustration 30: Spinal Twist

As you exhale, keep watching your hand as you swivel back to the starting place.

Take another inhalation, then exhale your way around to the right, again as far as you can.

As you're inhaling, notice what your fingertips are lined up with now. I'll bet the farm that you've gone farther than last time! Mentally mark the sport.

Exhale back to the starting position.

Go through the move two more times. Notice your progress each time and compare the last measurement to the first one. Congratulations!

Now go through the whole procedure on the other side, knees left, feet right, while watching the back of your right hand. Enjoy! Maybe you'd like to do a few more?

Compare how your back feels now to before you began. Are you impressed with how well your body responds to these gentle movements? Do you feel more lively and energetic? A little younger? I expect so!

When you continue practicing the Spiral Twist, you can add a more visual dimension to it. As you watch the back of your hand while you're twisting, move it toward your face and then back out. This way your lenses can get a limbering up as well.

VISUAL ADJUSTMENT

We're going to give your eyes something to read today, but it won't be letters yet. Let's put them through a series of preparatory warm-ups. First, notice your reading ability without glasses. Then take about five minutes for:

Three rounds of bouncing on the ball while counting colors in the room. Using your patch, work each eye separately and then both together.

Use your patch again for Picket Fence Swings. Tick-tick-tick back and forth with each eye, then both together. Last, close your eyes and mentally go over the fences again. Physically move your head and make the appropriate sound.

Move on to several minutes with your Spiral (or substitute the Finger Shift, including the step of watching the near finger come toward and away from your nose).

Next, turn back to the poem "Warning," and highlight the white between the lines and then around all the words. Does the print jump out clearly as you ignore it?

You've now loosened and expanded your vision, so we'll put this preparation to good use with the Number Bounce [illustration 31]. Music with a good beat, or a metronome, will keep your eyes nimble and the pace brisk as you shift your eyes rapidly through the numbers in sequence. Bounce on your ball for this.

Patch one eye, and have the page at a distance where you can see the largest numbers clearly without glasses.

Begin with the number 1, and let your eyes quickly move on through the numbers until you get to 50.

Breathe, blink, and trust your eyes to be drawn to the next

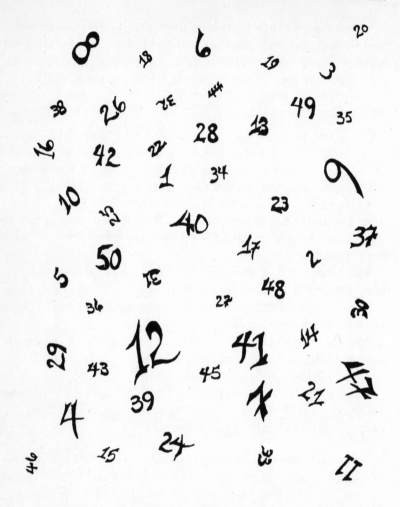

Illustration 31: Number Bounce

number, even if it's smaller than you think you can read. As with color counting, knowing what you're looking for enables your mind to boost the power of your vision.

When you get to 50, work your way back to one.

Next, move your patch to the other eye and repeat.

Then use both eyes together.

Finally, palm for ten long breaths.

Check your glasses-free reading ability again. Any difference?

As you work with this exercise, you may want to make a reduced copy of the numbers page. This way you can use them like the Near and Far Charts so you get even more of an accommodation workout. Of course, you would look from the 1 on the bigger page to the 1 on the small page, then the 2 on each one, and so forth.

TODAY

- Consciously explore an important past memory.
- Twist that spine—even if you're sitting in a chair.
- Do the Number Bounce again.
- Exercise your lenses with the Infinity Stretch.
- Take a Vision Walk.
- Sun on this walk.
- Be on the lookout for a good joke.
- Use the Chest Expansion to relax your shoulders and bring circulation into your eyes.

DAY TWENTY-SIX

Experience is not what happens to you, it is what you do with what happens to you.

Aldous Huxley
The Art of Seeing

ATTITUDE ADJUSTMENT

In 1910, sixteen-year-old Aldous Huxley was stricken with a severe case of keratitis, an inflammation of the cornea. He was nearly blind during this period, and when it subsided after eighteen months his corneas were covered with permanent scar tissue. By 1939, what little sight he had retained was deteriorating in spite of his use of the strongest possible glasses. The doctors told him there was no hope, that soon even what was left of his reading ability would go.

Huxley, however, heard about the Bates Method and became a student of Margaret Corbett, a legendary teacher of the techniques who entered the field after seeing it restore her husband's eyesight. Working intensively with Huxley, she helped him make use of and develop his remaining sight. While he had always deeply appreciated and used the vision he had rather than fall into despair over it, Corbett taught him visual skills and what he called "dynamic relaxation," which produced a relative miracle.

In *The Art of Seeing,* his book about his visual recovery, Huxley says, "Just as I was wondering apprehensively what on earth I should do, if reading were to become impossible, I happened to hear of a method of visual reeducation.... Within a couple of months I was reading without spectacles and, what was better still, without strain or fatigue."

His wife, Laura, details the extent of his visual independence in her beautiful memoir *This Timeless Moment: A Personal View of Aldous Huxley.* A man once dependent on others for nearly everything became able to travel throughout the world on his own. He was not only able to read without glasses, he was comfortable doing so for up to eight hours a day. He was intensely delighted by the details, colors, and textures of what he did see.

Whether it was conscious or subconscious, Huxley made a choice. He rejected misery over his impaired vision and opted instead for growth and discovery. He approached what others would call his handicap as a world to be explored with a sense of childlike wonder and curiosity. Seeing in a state of dynamic relaxation was for him to "be active, and yet remain relaxed; don't strain and yet do your damndest; stop trying so hard and let the deep-seated intelligence of your body and the subconscious mind do the work as it ought to be done."

In *Love, Medicine, and Miracles,* Dr. Bernie Siegel makes a strong case for a childlike attitude being one of the personality traits of survivors. I certainly see this in vision work as well. Childlike is very different, however, from childish. The former builds from experience; the latter whines about it. It is childlike to enter so deeply into flow experiences that one is unaware of all surrounding distractions. It's childish to focus on the distractions and be upset by them.

Citing the extensive research by psychologist Al Siebert, Siegel outlines an array of childlike attributes which indicate an ability to grow from life experiences. These include:

A sense of playfulness
A positive outlook, no matter the situation
Innocent curiosity
Total absorption in an activity
Being able to accept criticism
Taking mistakes in stride and being able to laugh about them
Good imagination
Nonconformity, yet not total rebellion
A sense that getting older means getting better and being able
    to enjoy yourself more

I really like that last one! It sure beats the alternative. From the standpoint of vision, it certainly makes sense that if you don't feel this way, your visual system will do you the favor of blurring out a perceived unpleasant reality. But the same reality, if perceived with love and acceptance, just naturally becomes more clear.

I know, easier said than done! There's good news, though. These survival traits can be learned by those of us who don't come by them naturally. The research shows it, and I certainly see it in myself and the people with whom I work. The most dramatic and delightful transformations most often occur during the course of residential workshops of a week or more. Not changes into something foreign, rather, a butterflylike emergence from a cocoon of dormant potential.

Far more often than not, the people who appear the least childlike and open at the start of workshops are the ones who step most fully into it. It takes some coaxing and prodding at first, but once they begin to enjoy the mental, physical, and visual experiences, there's no stopping them. They laugh the most and leave looking ten years younger and feeling in the springtime of their adulthood. These are generally my favorite people, perhaps because they encourage me in my own recurring moments of self-doubt.

But, hey, this is also a flow experience full of growth for me too. I have a good idea of what's coming, and I thoroughly enjoy every minute of it. Give me a room full of grim faces, and you've got a happy woman. My experience truly leads me to believe in our innate ability to manifest our full potential.

BREATHING AFFIRMATION

During the affirmation, perhaps you can entertain the idea of emerging free of any constrictions, like a butterfly from a cocoon. Consider the cocoon a safe place where you've been growing and gathering strength; now it's time to come out and fly.

Relax as you breathe from ten down to one. Affirm the following, or a phrase of your own, for at least ten more breaths:

Inhaling: "Willing to experience."

Exhaling: "Willing to grow."

Breathe up, using the image of spreading your wings and flying as you become more and more alert and energetic.

LIFESTYLE ADJUSTMENT

More spinal work is in store for today so as much circulation as possible will flow up into your ocular area. After you observe how you're feeling from head to toe, take at least five minutes with these preliminaries:

Begin with the Leg Lift Series, breathing deeply and noticing how it feels to do this today in comparison to the first time you did it.

Move on to Rolling Breaths. How do these feel compared to your first attempt?

Sit up and practice the Spinal Twist at least three times in each direction. How much improvement is there between the first and final rotations?

I took my first yoga lesson at the age of twenty-seven, while I was at the famous Rancho La Puerta health spa in Baja, California. The plush but often grueling weekend was my prize for an appearance on the television show *The Dating Game*. I was quite slender and looked to be the picture of health, but I was actually riddled with stress-related aches, pains, colds, and poor digestion.

I didn't know what yoga was, but it's slow gentleness appealed to me after a day of exhausting workouts. I quickly discovered, however, that I was appallingly stiff. It was especially apparent when I attempted the exercise you will learn today, the Spinal Stretch. My initial upward stretch was fine, but when I then tried to come forward and down over my knees, I went virtually nowhere. My spine was so rigid I was still in an upright position, and shooting pains ran up and down my back. If I was as "young as my spine was supple," I thought, I was seventy-two instead of twenty-seven!

The combination of my need for flexibility and the exquisite experience of the relaxation at the end of the class prompted me to join an ongoing class as soon as I returned home. Within a few weeks I could stretch out all the way over my legs in this posture, and within a year I was teaching classes. At twenty-eight, I was younger than I was the year before, and now, at fifty-one, my spine is more like that of a fifteen-year-old.

Be gentle with yourself as you work with your spine in this exercise. A series of slow easy moves is going to take you farther than a single intensive one, where you pull and strain to get into the right position. Remember the lesson on patience, and you'll see that it will help you progress far faster than will impatience and struggle.

As shown in illustration 32, begin sitting up with your legs stretched out in front of you. Inhale as you stretch up.

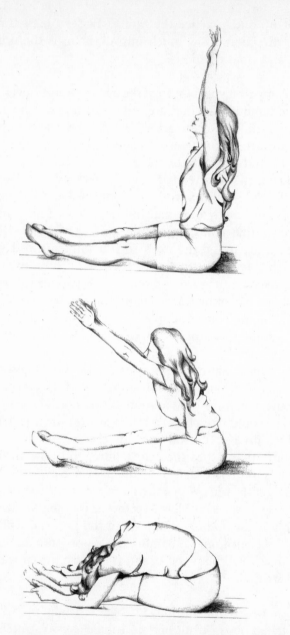

Illustration 32: Spinal Column Stretch

Hold your breath as you lean forward. You are reaching out and up with your arms, coming to a forty-five-degree angle over your legs.

Exhale as you stretch out and down over your legs. If there's no discomfort, pull yourself a little closer to your legs.

Hold the position for at least three easy breaths, letting yourself relax more into the stretch with each of your exhalations. Notice how far your head is from your knees—this is going to change for the better as you make this stretch a part of your life.

Repeat two more times. How much time do you have this morning? Can you do a few more repetitions?

How does your lower back feel? Hopefully, quite good. However, if it's a little strained, you were more than likely rounding it too much when you were stretched out over your legs. A round of Leg Lifts will relax it, and you can avoid a future occurrence by keeping your lower back flatter so the emphasis of your stretch is out and forward rather than down to your legs. Those smooth, easy repetitions are the key to coaxing your spine into flexibility.

VISUAL ADJUSTMENT

Before starting this session, take a look at the poem on pages 228–229, which is reproduced in three descending font sizes. Without glasses, how well can you read each one?

Today, there's another developmental reading-skill exercise, so put on some music and spend about five minutes warming up for it with:

String Fusion on the ball. Play with different speeds, sliding slowly from knot to knot and then as quickly as possible. How close to your nose can you bring your focus and still clearly see the strings crossing? How does this compare to your first try?

Massage whatever feels tense after the string work.
Palm for ten long whole-body breaths, more if necessary.
Keep your eyes closed and mentally do some Dot Swings.

Move your head as you imagine the black line moving in the opposite direction of your swing from dot to dot. Cover each of the four directions.

Play with the Spiral (or Picket Fence Swings) for a few minutes.

Now look at the three versions of the poem again. Any changes yet?

"The Salutation of the Day" was written in the fourth century A.D. by the Indian poet and playwright Kalidasa. This eloquent call to live in the present makes for excellent reading. As you work your way down through the three decreasing print sizes, by the end, or even on this first try, you may very well be able to read much smaller print than at the beginning.

For each step of the exercise, first use your patch to work each eye separately, and then use them together. Hold or place the page far enough away from you so that you can easily read the largest rendering of the poem.

First, use only the largest poem and at a comfortable distance where you can see it clearly.

Turn the book upside down and read the poem, one word at a time, from the last word at the bottom right corner back to the beginning. You're reading from right to left. Don't worry about content, just enjoy exploring the words and letters from this new perspective.

Do your eyes need a rest after this? If so, palm for ten to twenty breaths.

Turn the book right-side up again.

For the next steps of the exercise, go through all three sizes of the poem in descending order. Don't worry about whether or not you can see the print clearly.

First, scan back and forth along the white under each line.

Then continue keeping your head moving along with your eyes as you highlight the white around each word.

Move on to "shifting" on each word. Shift your gaze from the first letter of the word to the last, back and forth two times, before going on to the next. Don't worry about seeing them or the ones in between clearly, just shift from end to end. Breathe and blink!

Next, let your eyes jump over the words between the white spaces.

Now, skip the patching and read all the way through the poems. How does this compare to your initial reading?

Finally, massage around your eyes and then palm for twenty breaths.

TODAY

- What new experiences are you looking forward to?
- Stretch and twist your spine some more.
- Practice the reading lesson again.
- Scan a photo for details; memorize it and describe it.
- Give your lenses the Hot and Cold Treatment.
- Yawn and stretch in the sunshine.

The Salutation of the Day

Look to this day
For it is life.
The very life of life.
In its brief course lie
All the realities and verities of existence:
The bliss of growth,
The splendor of action,
The glory of power.
For yesterday is but a dream,
And tomorrow is only a vision,
But today, lived well,
Makes every yesterday a dream of
   happiness
And every tomorrow a vision of hope.
Look well therefore to this day.

The Salutation of the Day

Look to this day
For it is life.
The very life of life.
In its brief course lie
All the realities and verities of existence:
The bliss of growth,
The splendor of action,
The glory of power.
For yesterday is but a dream,
And tomorrow is only a vision,
But today, lived well,
Makes every yesterday a dream of happiness
And every tomorrow a vision of hope.
Look well therefore to this day.

The Salutation of the Day

Look to this day
For it is life.
The very life of life.
In its brief course lie
All the realities and verities of existence:
The bliss of growth,
The splendor of action,
The glory of power.
For yesterday is but a dream,
And tomorrow is only a vision,
But today, lived well,
Makes every yesterday a dream of happiness
And every tomorrow a vision of hope.
Look well therefore to this day.

DAY TWENTY-SEVEN

> Intention is the active partner of attention, it is the
> way we convert automatic processes to conscious ones.
>
> Deepak Chopra
> *Ageless Body, Timeless Mind*

ATTITUDE ADJUSTMENT

To get the most out of the attention you now pay to your vision
and the exercises you do to improve it, your intention must stay
clear and focused. This sounds simple, and, indeed, it is at its
core, but most of us have an established habit of losing sight of
our real goals and operating on the half steam of automatic
pilot. Going through the motions, without attention backed up
by the directing force of intention wastes an enormous amount
of time and energy.

The same principle applies to everything we do, but it's
especially crucial when the aim is healing and a change in habit
or thought patterns. Quantity without quality won't do the job,
and what constitutes quality can be very different for each
individual. This is why "scientific" data on vision improvement
and other applications of mind-and-body healing is so sketchy.
Healing and inner changes take place in a realm still beyond the
measuring ability of science.

As sketchy as the scientific evidence is, it's certainly not
nonexistent. It has been demonstrated, for example, that something as straightforward as physical fitness can be highly affected by the quality of attention and intention. Of course,
performance is improved by a positive expectation and focused
concentration, but it still appears that greater changes in areas
like muscle mass and bone density occur when they are clearly
kept in mind as primary intentions. It's not an achievement of
mind over matter, it's one of mind *with* matter.

When it comes to vision work, the obvious overriding intention is to see clearly. However, the more this general intention is
broken down and defined, the more efficiently our brain can
send out all the right instructions for the desired changes. So,

several questions must be asked, such as, what do you want to see clearly? The printed page, right? But of course, you can't have selective near vision; it's an all or nothing proposition. Are you willing to accept a clear view of *everything* up close? Including yourself?

What's more, can you go beyond acceptance and draw from the emotional quality that is the very essence of healing power? This is, naturally, love. It encompasses love for yourself (including every sign of age), your eyes, and the precious power of sight. Has the experience of relating to your eyes as beloved twin babies in need of loving healing stayed with you since the first week of the program? Focusing on this as your intention is worth weeks of mechanical shifting back and forth between the Near and Far Charts.

Which brings us to what I suppose would be called a sub-intention. The overall goal of restoring clarity through loving intention is best achieved when the exercises become flow experiences. These, we know, happen most often when we are engaged in the art of enjoying something for its own sake rather than the end product or result. While working in Germany, I learned a word for this which I think brings good energy to any activity with the potential of slipping into meaningless rote mechanics: *Funktionlust*!

Funktionlust actually translates into what I assume Mihaly Csikszentmihalyi would accept as a definition of enjoyment, as it means "the pleasure of doing." Clearly, the German *lust* took on its sexual and greedy connotations when we incorporated it into the English language! Still, I find the juxtaposition of the dry and the passionate in *Funktionlust* a delight. A lusty approach will definitely elevate a mere "function" to a far more interesting level.

Our larger intention to restore clarity through loving healing now takes on the aspect of continual freshness. Again, however, we can be even more specific. Involvement in each moment of every exercise should carry with it a true expectation of clarity. This means, for example, that while the benefits of the near-and-far chartwork are cumulative, each shift to near-point has the potential to produce immediate clearing. If we don't pay attention to this possibility, as well as to the enjoyment of the activity, we may actually miss it when it happens.

This is one of the reasons I have stressed always looking at a printed page without glasses before automatically resorting to them. I was not aware that people even did this until Jim Newberry, my bodyworker extraordinaire, started catching himself putting them on when he didn't really need them. When a highly aware individual does this, it shows just how insidious our habitual programming can be.

In fact, this in-the-moment kind of guy even displayed the all-too-human lack of positive expectation during his initial step back from presbyopia. It was the first time I introduced him to vision work. I had a Fusion String handy (I keep one in my purse), so we played with it while I explained a few basics. Afterward, we were sitting very close together as we talked. When he looked at me, I instantly realized two things: he could see me perfectly clearly (indicated by a sparkle in the eyes as if a veil has been lifted), and he wasn't consciously aware of it. I zapped him with the facts, and had my laugh fest of the day when his expression lit up to match his eyes. And so began our working partnership.

The intention of expectation applies as much to aging as it does to vision. Dr. Chopra expresses it well: "The decline of vigor in old age is largely the result of people *expecting* to decline; they have unwittingly implanted a self-defeating intention in the form of a strong belief, and the body-mind connection automatically carries out this intention."

ATTITUDE ADJUSTMENT

Expect a relaxing and positive experience! Breathe your way down from ten to one, and affirm for the next ten breaths:

Inhaling: "Clear intentions."

Exhaling: "Clear sight."

After you've counted up, alert and refreshed, begin to think about your intentions, specifically, for your vision and for the kind of day you would like this to become.

LIFESTYLE ADJUSTMENT

Jump right in to setting a good mood for the day with a few good laughs!

Laugh silently with your mouth open.
Laugh silently with your mouth closed.
Laugh out loud at yourself!

Release more tension with:

Yoga Neck Stretches
Kinesthetic Swings
Stretching, and Curling Up and Down

Let's take the concept of optimism and positive expectation into the practical Lifestyle Adjustment of Mental Rehearsal. We're all great at mental rehearsal, we do it all the time. Unfortunately, an awful lot of us have the tendency to get it backward. We dwell on what could go wrong, and, what a surprise, that's often just what happens. We worry about things we can't change, draining our very life force and reinforcing the negative outcome.

Not all of us, of course. When the traits of highly successful individuals are studied, one that consistently turns up is the rehearsal, rather than just the projection, of excellent performance and positive outcomes. These are people in every walk of life, though to most of us the best known are usually sports figures. Florence Griffith Joyner, for example, attributes her Olympic gold medals and record-breaking speed as much to her mental work as to her rigorous training regimen. She spent more time listening to motivational tapes and visualizing each detail of her upcoming races than she did on the track.

Down here on the earthly level, it's still true that success, health, and well-being go hand in hand with considering what is ahead and then mentally projecting an ideal, yet attainable, outcome. "Attainable" is a key word here, meaning the height of optimistic realism, the best possible case scenario. Considering what is ahead is also key. Plans should be flexible, but making them creates a clear focus of intention to guide our attitudes and actions.

Today you have an opportunity to create a mental spring-board for both optimal vision and personal satisfaction. The rehearsal experiences is laid out as a visualization, but if visual imagery doesn't come easily to you, don't struggle with it. As long as your mind is in a positive mode anyway, it will play with the possibilities.

It's not imperative, but Palming while you envision a day of clear (or clearer) vision and smooth sailing through life's tides will give you an extra boost in vision. Read over the scripted guidelines, then close your eyes and create your own attainable ideal day.

Begin by counting five slow whole-body breaths. Feel yourself expanding gently with the breaths in, and relaxing more deeply with each breath out.

Imagine waking up in the morning feeling refreshed and looking forward to your day. See yourself, your bed, the room, and anyone who shares it with you. If there's someone else there, give him or her the same positive attitude.

Even before you get out of bed, consider the day ahead and plan accordingly. What are your goals? What do you need to do to accomplish them?

See yourself getting up, stretching, yawning, and energizing with some of your favorite exercises. Make a few of them specifically for your vision. How about a few laughs?

Go over your regular morning routine, envisioning every-thing going smoothly and pleasantly.

Even if you don't generally read in the morning, let a newspaper, book, or magazine be in this picture. What is it? Imagine reading the print easily without glasses, or, if that is completely unrealistic at this point, with a much weaker prescription.

As you imagine reading, visualize the act of reading as well as the print itself (how about: "Today, well lived, makes every yesterday a dream of happiness and every tomorrow a vision of hope").

Picture the rest of your day unfolding. See the everyday tasks as a source of pleasure and accomplishment. Experience your interactions with other people as compatible and mutually satisfying. See yourself as confident and optimistic, full of life and energy.

Allow an image of something not happening as you would have wanted. See yourself adapting, knowing this situation is not personal, permanent, or pervasive. You can deal with difficulties. You can bounce back!

Every now and then, include reading material in the details of your day. Rehearse the pleasures of having and maintaining clearer sight. See yourself taking a few minutes here and there to revitalize your vision, mind, and body. Which exercises would you choose?

Shouldn't this day include a Vision Walk in the sunshine? Where would this be the most pleasant? Picture and feel yourself indulging in Sunning.

As your daytime activities wind down, move on to creating a realistically ideal evening. Include some reading in it!

Go all the way through to the conclusion of your evening. Rehearse caring for yourself and your vision, sharing with those in your life, enjoying meaningful activities.

You finally drift off to sleep, contented, fulfilled, and looking forward to tomorrow.

When you're ready, stretch and yawn, and know you can make this (flexible) vision a reality!

Make positive and productive mental rehearsal a regular habit! There's nothing in your life that can't benefit from it, whether it's daily life or a particular goal or skill.

VISUAL ADJUSTMENT

Warm up for today's reading lesson for at least five minutes divided among the following exercises. If you prefer to concentrate your time on just a couple, that's certainly fine too.

The Hot and Cold Treatment
Infinity Stretch
Finger Shift, on the ball, followed by Palming
Spiral (or String Fusion)

Okay, time to read. As you can see, each of the following sentences is reproduced in five descending font sizes. The reading skill directions, all of which you already know, are contained in the sentences themselves. They also serve as affirmations and suggestions to reinforce these skills at the subconscious level.

Take a look at the first sentence in the exercise. Can you already read all five diminishing lines without glasses? If so, be sure to do the exercise anyway. It's a perfect maintenance routine.

If you can't see all the lines clearly, take note of how many you can. Expect this number to increase during the session as you follow the instructions and make use of one of your most powerful tools for changing your vision—your memory.

When you come to a line you can't read, look back to the one you can. Memorize it, noticing all the curves and angles of the letters.

Then close your eyes and remember it. See it clearly in your mind's eye, especially the contrast between the black and white. Imagine the print as smaller than it appeared, but just as clear.

Then open your eyes again and look down to the line that had just been blurry. It may clear for you immediately, or it may take a little practice before your memory stimulates a visual response. It will!

This is one of the exercises many of my clients like to go over before starting their "real" reading. Warming up before reading, just like stretching before running, enhances comfort and performance. Experiment to find out what works best for you. It could be anything from a preliminary reading exercise to a good Facial Massage or a rousing round of Finger Shifts.

I am interested only in highlighting the
whiteness as I slide my eyes under the lines
of print.

I am interested only in highlighting the whiteness as I
slide my eyes under the lines of print.

I am interested only in highlighting the whiteness as I slide
my eyes under the lines of print.

I am interested only in highlighting the whiteness as I slide my eyes under the
lines of print.

I am interested only in highlighting the whiteness as I slide my eyes under the lines of print.

When I read I am most aware of the white
under and around the words and letters.

When I read I am most aware of the white under and
around the words and letters.

When I read I am most aware of the white under and around
the words and letters.

When I read I am most aware of the white under and around the words and
letters.

When I read I am most aware of the white under and around the words and letters.

As I remain aware of white, the black print
stands out in clear contrast.

As I remain aware of white, the black print stands out
in clear contrast.

As I remain aware of white, the black print stands out in clear
contrast.

As I remain aware of white, the black print stands out in clear contrast.

As I remain aware of white, the black print stands out in clear contrast.

The more I practice seeing the letters clearly in my mind, the more easily I can read a printed page.

The more I practice seeing the letters clearly in my mind, the more easily I can read a printed page.

The more I practice seeing the letters clearly in my mind, the more easily I can read a printed page.

The more I practice seeing the letters clearly in my mind, the more easily I can read a printed page.

The more I practice seeing the letters clearly in my mind, the more easily I can read a printed page.

My lenses are flexible, and I can read clearly up-close.

My lenses are flexible, and I can read clearly up-close.

My lenses are flexible, and I can read clearly up-close.

My lenses are flexible, and I can read clearly up-close.

My lenses are flexible, and I can read clearly up-close.

TODAY

- Remember that it is your intention to see clearly as you exercise your eyes, not just to go through repetitive motions.
- Before any special encounters or activities (including reading), rehearse a positive outcome.
- Read a paragraph upside down and backwards.
- Practice highlighting white and reading descending print sizes.
- Notice if you're tight anywhere on your head, face, neck or shoulders. Massage there!
- Count colors wherever you go.
- Play with the Fusion String or the Spiral.
- Yawn!

DAY TWENTY-EIGHT

Quit acting your age!

Bodyworker/Healer Jim Newberry to Lisette Scholl

ATTITUDE ADJUSTMENT

Jim zaps me with that one very now and then. Easy for him to say, he hasn't reached fifty yet! Actually, I used to take great pride in never having acted my age, at least once I was over twenty-one. However, I'm changing my attitude. I've decided I like my age, and I like acting it. That's because I perceive it and the aging process differently than I did a few years ago. I no longer feel young for someone in her fifties; I feel that as someone in her fifties, I am young.

Being fifty is not what is was one hundred, fifty, or even ten years ago. Whatever your age, the same applies. We are biologically younger at the same age than generations before us. We don't have to work out incessantly at the gym to claim what's already our birthright. All we have to do is make a shift in our consciousness. We don't need to become younger, but just to realize how young we are.

For all the talk about the rejuvenation of your eyes, I want to stress their current youth. They have evolved along with the rest of the human body, but negative conditioning has impeded the development of their full potential. In some ways, it's as simple as the way we treat our teeth. If we don't take care of them, they don't last much longer than the caveman's, but give them a little brushing and flossing and they can go the distance.

Of course, vision improvement is far more complex, especially when it's bound to our attitudes about aging. Still, it's simply embracing the enormous positive potential of both vision and age that's at the heart of achieving them. When you consider the alternative, why not?

The quotations and affirmations this and every week of our workshop embody life-affirming concepts that can bring our potential into reality. As you look through them and breathe along with the affirmations, be aware of how true they ring for you.

1. "Joy and fulfillment keep us healthy and extend life."
   Inhaling: "I choose"
   Exhaling: "Joy and fulfillment."

2. "Do not take life too seriously. You will never get out of it alive."
   Inhaling: "I choose"
   Exhaling: "Laughter and joy."

3. "Jonathan Livingston Seagull discovered that boredom and fear and anger are the reasons a gull's life is so short, and with these gone from his thought, he lived a fine long life indeed."
   Inhaling: "To enjoy"
   Exhaling: "Is to live."

4. "When we acknowledge the comedy of time, we recover the power of memory. Like time, memory can be recovered at any point and brought into the eternal now. Like time, too, all its strands and forces can be gathered for the edification of the present. If you have lost or blocked your memories, chances are you have also blocked or lost the times of your life."
   Inhaling: "Remembering the past."
   Exhaling: "Clearing the present."

5. "Experience is not what happens to you, it is what you do with what happens to you."
   Inhaling: "Willing to experience."
   Exhaling: "Willing to grow."

6. "Intention is the active partner, it is the way we convert automatic processes to conscious ones."
   Inhaling: "Clear intentions."
   Exhaling: "Clear sight."

Which one draws you in the most? Spend five more breaths on it.

This could be good regular practice. All the affirmations in the book are always available to you as attitudinal lifts whenever you are in need of one. Creating your own, of course, may be even more effective. Whichever your chose, this conscious focusing of intention is a habit we can all benefit from.

LIFESTYLE ADJUSTMENT

I'm curious as to which of the vast array of lifestyle exercises you've learned will become an ongoing part of your life. Which have the most immediate visual benefits? Are they also favorite exercises of yours, or do you enjoy others more? It's good to pay attention to what you deem especially beneficial, but don't let it get in the way of the enjoyment factor. It boosts benefits and keeps you coming back. Again, I stress Edgar Cayce's maxim: "The best exercises for you are the ones you will do."

Can you recall how far down you could curl and how comfortable this stretch felt on the first day? If we are "as young as the spine is supple," how much younger are you now? Which stretches feel the best?

The most fundamental of all the exercises and lifestyle habits has to be breathing. If you still catch yourself tightening or holding your breath regularly, persevere! Every deeper breath revitalizes you, as does each glass of water and bite of nutritional food. Don't waste your vital energy regretting other choices, build it by savoring your successes. Spend it on the expansion of enjoyment in your life!

The research, you'll remember, breaks the effects of enjoyment down into two different but equally important types. Regularly occurring episodes of moderate pleasure and enjoyment are most associated with longevity. Bursts of out-and-out hilarity and wild joy, on the other hand, provide immediate release of internal chemicals which produce pain-free euphoria, stress release, and physical healing responses. Clearly, the best combination is an ongoing optimistic interpretation of life seasoned with occasional doses of glee. Sounds good to me.

Let's start with that spice of life, laughter, as we review the week's lifestyle exercises. Take a few moments before you close your eyes and observe your body and sense of well-being as they are right now.

Begin with laughing. If at all possible, do this while looking in a mirror! Do thirty seconds or more each of Silent Laughing With Mouth Closed, Silent Laughing With Mouth Open, an out loud Ha-Ha-Ha, and Ho-Ho-Ho. How do you feel now?

Your chest and shoulders are primed to open and relax more, so move onto a Chest Expansion. Hold the bent forward position for three or four long breaths. Feel more open afterward? The circulation in your face and eyes?

Now sit down and sense your spine and back muscles at this point. Loosen and stretch them with Spinal Twists, three in each direction. Gauge your progress by noticing where your fingers line up with background objects. Twist around on your exhalations. Appreciate your mobility and the increased comfort in your back.

Elongate your spine as you stretch your back and legs with the Spinal Stretch. Hold the stretch over your legs for a few breaths, and then relax and curl back up into the starting position. Do this three times.

Bring your attention to your face and eyes. Check your reading ability without glasses. See what changes you feel and see after indulging in several minutes of the Accupressure Massage.

This completes the review of this week's physical exercise introductions. Did it serve as a good overall session for you? Would you feel even better with more stretching and breathing?

If so, you have many choices. I'd probably tend toward the Leg Lift Series and/or Rocking Breaths and Rolling Breaths, but follow your instincts!

Compare how you feel now to before you began.

Relax, close your eyes, and spend several minutes visualizing your ideal attainable day. See everything going right for all concerned. Experience reading print easily, and fitting good nutrition, water, stretching, a few vision exercises, and a lot of laughter into your day. What else is in your ideal scenario? Follow it to its conclusion before yawning and stretching into alertness.

Taking the time for a series of exercises that build upon each other is ideal, but every little stretch and deeper-than-normal breath counts, and positive expectation counts. Small adjustments in your daily routine are equally, if not more, important than set-aside workout times.

VISUAL ADJUSTMENT

For a certain viewpoint, this is the bottom line: How much improvement has there been in your near-point clarity since you began the Totally Timeless Program? Are you free of reading glasses, more independent, using a weaker prescription?

If you've actually been able to devote concentrated time and effort to this project for twenty-eight days in a row and move straight through it, I'm impressed! I'll admit, even more than when we started out, that this is a feat I wouldn't expect of many. If you've done it, I fervently hope the rewards are well worth the effort. If they haven't met your expectations, let me make a few points. These actually apply to everyone, regardless of how long you've stretched out the program.

Unless you were only mildly presbyopic to begin with, twenty-eight days can actually be considered a remarkably quick recovery time. The combination of long-term habits, beliefs, attitudes, and expectations, along with years of dormancy and poor nutrition, can take longer than a few weeks to reverse.

If you've quickly come a long way, congratulations, but, once again, equal kudos for however far you've progressed! Further rejuvenation will accompany that now finely honed skill of patient perseverance. Guidelines for the continuing quest, as well as the maintenance of what you have achieved, are in the concluding chapter. Meanwhile, let's go over this weeks vision exercises so you can better integrate them into your continuing visual development.

Before you begin, gauge your present near-point clarity

again. Check it at the end of each exercise, and you'll have a better idea if any are particularly stimulating to your close vision. Play your favorite rhythmic mood music.

Begin by loosening up your near vision with Picket Fence Swings. Spend about a minute using all three sizes of fences with your eyes open. Then one more minutes with your eyes closed. Continue to move your head as you imagine running your stick back and forth over a tiny fence suspended about fourteen inches in front of your face.

Next, turn to the "When I Am an Old Woman I Will Wear Purple" reading page. Highlight the white back and forth under every line of print.

Now let your eyes run rapidly through the white trail through the Labyrinth and then back again to the beginning.

Keep them moving at a quick pace through the Number Chart from 1 to 50 and back again. Breathe and blink!

Work next with the three sizes of "Salutation to The Day." First turn the book upside down and read the largest print backward from the lower right corner all the way back to the upper left.

Finally, use the fifth reading-affirmation sentence in Day twenty-seven: "My lenses are flexible and I can read clearly up close."

Position the book so the first and largest line of print is clear. Can you read any of the other lines as well? The first one you cannot see clearly will be the one you'll work with.

Take a good look at the larger "My." Memorize it. Close your eyes and remember it clearly and *smaller*. Open them and look at the smaller "My." Do this with each word of the sentence.

The smaller versions of each word should start coming in more clearly as you work your way through them. If it's not happening yet—practice, practice!

Now give your eyes a good rest. They would love five minutes or more of Palming, but do what you can. Then give them a final pick-me-up by massaging around them and on your eyebrows and forehead.

How did this workout affect your vision? How do the results compare with those from even more strenuous exercises like String Fusion and the Finger Shift? With more Sunning and massage? With the Spiral and the Hot and Cold Treatments? From now on, I cannot say which exercises are the best for you, this must be your decision. I'll offer ideas, but let your instincts and occasional browsing back through all the review days guide your choices.

TODAY

- What affirmation (quite possibly one of your own making) sums up what you want to focus on at this point?
- How many Lifestyle Adjustments have slipped into your daily routine? A regular ongoing practice session?
- How do you use your eyes differently than you did a month ago? In what ways do you feel differently about them?
- What are the little things you regularly do to keep your vision as sharp as can be?
- Use the last chapter to plan your future vision care.

PART TWO

FUTURE VISION

FUTURE VISION

Paradoxical as it may seem; to believe in youth is to
look backward, to look forward we must believe in age.

Dorothy L. Sayers

We are incredibly lucky to be part of the Age Wave, the
worldwide post–World War II baby boom which boasts nearly
seventy-seven million members in the United States alone. We
will not have to muster the individual courage it has taken to age
well, especially in our youth obsessed culture. A mass movement
often likened to "a pig moving through a python," we are a force
of nature just reaching its crest. No other group has the power to
tell us how to age—we're in control here.

In the concluding lines of *The Age Wave*, Ken Dychtwald sums
up our future potential by saying, "The Age Wave will give us
not merely the opportunity to live well and to live long, drawing
much from life, but will also provide us with the time and energy
to give more back, enriching society and ourselves with the
special qualities and deep experiences of long life."

Once our youth obsession transcends into an embrace of our
maturity and the fact of its unprecedented longevity, we can
recover from the grip of what has been a sort of premature
cultural presbyopia. We haven't been willing to see and accept
many of the signs of our aging. However, we'll bounce right back
from this denial as we fully comprehend the new frontier ahead,
one that was never available to past generations. The exponen-

tial leaps in evolution, consciousness, and technology in the few centuries since the Renaissance will look primitive by comparison.

I know, there are all kinds of pitfalls and disasters we may encounter or wreak. Certainly we need to take care and make precautions, but, just as with any attitudinal outlook, it's the positive expectations that most promote positive outcomes. We have a choice of attitudes toward the future. Why not choose the most optimistic one?

Remember when I mentioned the astronomical event on January 23, 1997, that could be interpreted as the heralding of our entry into the Age of Aquarius, the ultimate renaissance? Due to an unforeseen editing opportunity on this book, I can report that I actually saw a sign of confirmation. At the worldwide appointed time I read a Native American prayer and then looked down at a small and special valley below. To my utter astonishment, a large rainbow materialized seventy-five feet away, emanating from the branches of a large oak tree and arcing into the center of the meadow. I hadn't asked for a sign, but I certainly chose to know one when I saw it!

In twenty-five or thirty years, when I may begin to slow down a little, I plan to be looking out over that same valley, or a similar one deeper in the countryside. What I envision there at that time is a retirement community far different than anything my parents' generation could dream of. What do you expect as your lifestyle for the last ten years or so of your life? Do you know that experiments in elevating our later years beyond aimless leisure and survival are already well under way? We'll have more comfort, but we'll also have boundless opportunities to continue growing until we die. We will not be warehoused; we'll be "elderheroes."

Communities geared toward golf and a few other leisure activities are already well established. As they continue to expand, however, a number of "lifestyle towns" centered around historical interests have sprung up, in which residents create and live in reproductions of specific eras and locales. This trend of matching lifestyles to interests is expanding rapidly. Ken Dychtwald projects that it won't be long before there are communities for the sports-minded, fitness buffs, seekers of psychological and spiritual self-development, the horticulturally oriented, technotypes, and those dedicated to ongoing travel experiences.

This is an exciting list, though Dychtwald didn't include my projected back-to-the-land, self-sufficient commune made up of creative craftspeople and practitioners of the healing arts. The possibilities are as endless as the avenues we choose for self-expression and development. What ideal attainable future do you project?

One of my predictions about the future of vision care is that in less than ten years you will have a choice of methods to reverse your presbyopia. This one will still be available, but I have no doubt that there will also be the option of surgical implantation. When a market of nearly seventy-seven million presbyopes in this country alone becomes disgruntled with the annoyance of glasses, you can bet that the wizards of optical science and medicine will come up with a solution.

What if you had this choice today? Knowing what you know now, would you have passed up this chance to explore your visual and aging processes in depth? There will be a maintenance or continued improvement plan in your future. Can you see it as a vehicle for overall mind-and-body fitness as well? There are many paths to continued growth, and we can travel a variety of them at the same or at different times. It seems only natural to have one which includes the integration of our most vital sensory perception.

Consider the holistic benefits you'd gain from the following example of a possible ongoing visual maintenance program:

As you awaken, you yawn mightily and stretch lazily. As you get up, you turn on some pleasant and rhythmic music.

For five or ten minutes, you stretch through your entire body in time to the music. This morning you enjoy Rocking Breaths, then Rolling Breaths, and, finally, the Leg Lift Series.

Sitting up, you give yourself a quick but thorough Facial Massage. Now it's time for your shower, during which your scenario for the ideal attainable day runs (visually) through your mind.

Afterward, you dress to the entertainment of a cartoon program on TV, laughing heartily at it and the faces you make at your reflection in the mirror.

On with the day! While walking or driving from place to place you enjoy breathing deeply, noticing colors and details, and yawning. If the sun is out, you briefly bathe your closed eyes in it as often as possible. During your regular activities you take a brief break at least every hour. A little stretching, curling up and down, a Chest Expansion, and you're refreshed, ready to go again.

Whenever you read, you remember to breathe, blink, and let your eyes relax along the whiteness rather than strain over the print. After every second or third page you look into the distance, then rapidly in and out a half dozen more times before resuming reading. If your eyes feel at all tired, you palm and massage.

Let's say you've been noticing that it takes longer to focus clearly on your near point. You decide to counteract this for a week with several daily five-minute workouts with the Fusion String while bouncing on the ball, followed by a Hot and Cold Treatment.

Your food today favors healthy choices for the most part. Supplements make up for transgressions and extra needs, and sipping your way through a glass of water every hour or so is routine.

As your day gives way into its evening routine, you take ten minutes to rejuvenate mentally, physically, and visually. Today you do Long Swings to the Pachelbel Canon in D, the Crocodile, and palm for ten breaths to the Breathing Affirmation "Refreshing, Relaxing." Finally, you tune up your near-point vision and set your mood for the evening by reading through and seeing if you have any of the Symptoms of Inner Peace (see page 254).

There's something for the continual regeneration of every part of you in these small adjustments to daily life. Out of this vast handbook of possibilities I've supplied, you can mix and match according to your own preferences and needs. A little here and there will keep your vision sharp and give you plenty of time for the major joys and challenges in this phase of your life.

When I think of what else makes life good and vision clear I come up with three simple words: fun, touch, and love. Simple words, profound secrets of youthfulness. Don't overlook the regenerating and healing power of touch. We know babies don't thrive without it, did we think that changed as we age? There is enormous therapeutic value (including visual) from massage, chiropractic, and other bodywork, but it is the human factor that's the most rejuvenating.

To see clearly, stay in touch, have fun, and love what's closest to you!

THE PEACE PILGRIM'S SYMPTOMS
OF INNER PEACE

1. A tendency to think and act spontaneously rather than from fear based on past experiences

2. An unmistaken ability to enjoy each moment

3. Loss of interest in judging other people

4. Loss of interest in judging yourself

5. Loss of interest in interpreting the actions of others

6. Loss of interest in conflict

7. Loss of ability to worry (a very serious symptom)

8. Frequent, overwhelming episodes of appreciation

9. Contented feelings of connectedness with others and nature

10. Frequent attacks of smiling through the eyes from the heart

11. An increasing tendency to let things happen rather than make them happen

12. Increased susceptibility to love extended by others as well as the uncontrollable urge to extend it

RECOMMENDED READING

Belsky, Janet K. *Here Tomorrow: Making the Most of Life After Fifty.* Baltimore: Johns Hopkins Univ. Press, 1988.

Chopra, Deepak. *Ageless Body, Timeless Mind.* Harmony Books, 1993.

Cousins, Norman. *Anatomy of an Illness.* New York: W. W. Norton, 1979.

Csikszentmihalyi, Mihaly. *Flow: The Psychology of Optimal Experience.* New York: Harper and Row, 1990.

Dychtwald, Ken. *The Age Wave.* New York: J. P. Tarcher, 1989.

Dyer, Wayne. *You'll See It When You Believe It.* New York: Avon Books, 1990.

Earle, Richard, and David Imrie. *Your Vitality Quotient.* New York: Warner Books, 1989.

Goleman, Daniel. *Emotional Intelligence: Why It Can Matter More Than I.Q.* New York: Bantam Books, 1995.

Hendler, Sheldon Saul. *The Oxygen Breakthrough: 30 Days to an Illness-Free Life.* New York: Morrow, 1989.

Hendricks, Gay. *Conscious Breathing.* New York: Bantam Books, 1995.

Houston, Jean. *The Possible Human.* New York: J. P. Tarcher, 1982.

Huxley, Aldous. *The Art of Seeing.* Montana Books, 1975.

Huxley, Laura. *This Timeless Moment: A Personal View of Aldous Huxley.* Celestial Arts, 1975.

Kabat-Zinn, Jon. *Full Catastrophe Living.* New York: Dell Publishing, 1990.

Kaplan, Robert-Michael. *Seeing Without Glasses.* New York: Beyond Words Pub., 1994.

Liberman, Jacob. *Take Off Your Glasses and See*. New York: Crown Trade Paperback, 1995.

Leonard, George, and Michael Murphy. *The Life We Are Given*. New York: G. P. Putnam's Sons, 1995.

Levine, Barbara. *Your Body Believes Every Word You Say*. Aslan Publishing, 1991.

Leviton, Richard. *Brain Builders! A Lifelong Guide to Sharper Thinking, Better Memory, and an Age-Proof Mind*. Parker Publishing, 1995.

McWilliams, John Roger and Peter McWilliams. *You Can't Afford the Luxury of a Negative Thought*. Prelude Press, 1988.

Ott, John. *Health and Light*. New York: Pocket Books, 1976.

Pearsall, Paul. *The Pleasure Prescription*. Hunter House, 1996.

―――. *Super Joy: Learning to Celebrate Everyday Life*. New York: Doubleday, 1988.

Pogrebin, Letty Cottin. *Getting Over Getting Older*. Little Brown, 1996.

Schneider, Meir. *The Handbook of Self-Healing*. Arkana Penguin Books, 1994.

―――. *Self-Healing: My Life and Vision*. Routledge and Kegan Paul, 1987.

Scholl, Lisette. *Hypnovision: The Natural Way to Vision Improvement*. New York: Henry Holt, 1990.

―――. *Visionetics: The Holistic Way to Better Eyesight*. New York: Doubleday/Dolphin, 1978.

Seligman, Martin. *Learned Optimism*. New York: Alfred A. Knopf, 1990.

Sheey, Gail. *New Passages: Mapping Your Life Across Time*. New York: Ballantine Books, 1995.

Siegel, Bernie. *Love, Medicine, and Miracles*. New York: Harper and Row, 1986.